Patient Testimonials

"Doctor Goswami was such a great find as I was at the point of giving up my cherished trail running and climbing pursuits. Well after two stem cell treatments I am back at it, and am looking forward to many more years of joy. I greatly appreciated the care he took explaining in detail the procedure, the care in execution, and the many caring follow up calls. He is the best! We are excited that many more will learn and gain more knowledge about stem cells through this wonderful book."
    —*Megan and Paul Stevenson*

"Fascinating read. As a successful recipient of stem cell treatment for my shoulder, it was very rewarding to learn about the science behind *The Stem Cell Cure*. I highly recommend this book to anyone who would love to stay active and avoid surgery."
    —*Eric Davidson, Owner of Orange County Breakers*
    and World Team Tennis

"I tore my entire knee playing football in college and was trending toward replacement. The stem cell procedure was a breeze. After six months, I could see regrown cartilage with improvements in motion. I knew there had to be a better route than cutting myself open again with another surgery. This book helps distill important concepts of stem cell therapy, I recommend it to every athlete and non-athlete."
    —*Michael Spanos II, Los Angeles Chargers*

THE
STEM CELL
CURE

THE
STEM CELL
CURE

REMAKE YOUR
BODY AND YOUR MIND

GAURAV GOSWAMI, M.D.
KERRY JOHNSON, Ph.D.

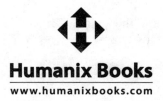

Humanix Books

www.humanixbooks.com

To Nimi and Sanju

Your silence has taught me more than any words could ever.

—GG

To Cora

My first grandchild and the light of my life.

—KJ

"The body is a cell state in which every cell is a citizen. Disease is merely the conflict of the citizens of the state brought about by the action of external forces" and "every cell arises from another cell."

—Rudolf Virchow, 1821–1902
Physician, Pathologist, and
Anthropologist

Contents

Preface

From the turn of the century, stem cells have been a burning topic. That will continue for the next several years. With anything new comes a whole range of opinions—responses that may or may not be rooted in the facts. Stem cells are making news, sometimes for the right reasons and other times for the wrong reasons. There are advocates who swear by stem cells and groups that denounce them. All of this can get very confusing for you, the consumer. How do you separate fact from fiction? That was the underlying motivation in deciding to write this book. We have tried to present the foundations as you consider stem cell treatments. We will address various conditions that can potentially be helped with stem cell treatments. Unlike other books on stem cells, we have tried to be as objective as possible. We don't advocate a particular type of treatment. Our goal is to provide you with as comprehensive an introduction to the world of stem cells as possible.

Nikola Tesla championed electromagnetic theory. But it took years to apply that discovery to cell phones and electric transportation. A similar revolution in medicine is taking place. In technology, the basic concepts of physics were discovered long ago. In medicine we have also known for as long that the fundamental units of our body are cells. It's at the cellular level that things go wrong. This ultimately manifests in disease. We have over-used pharmaceuticals and complicated surgeries to fix our health. While both of these have and will continue to play a role in certain conditions, the majority of our day-to-day medical needs can be addressed without them.

Introducing the Authors

It is rare for a physician and his patient to join hands and write about their experiences. One author was a patient and the other his physician. From two different vantage points, we hope you will get a balanced view of where things stand. For the physician in the book, Dr. Goswami, the journey has spread across continents, clinics, hospitals, university medical centers, and specialties. Dr. Goswami is cross-trained in both surgery and then interventional radiology. These trainings complement each other. While the role of a surgeon is clear, that of an interventional radiologist is often poorly understood. Unlike the radiologists who read imaging studies such as X-rays, CT scans, MRIs, or mammograms, interventional radiologists perform minimally invasive procedures using imaging guidance. Utilizing X-ray, ultrasound, and CT guidance allows them to offer techniques beyond open surgery.

A surgeon at heart, Dr. Goswami embraced the mindset that a surgeon dies with his scrubs on. The underlying guiding principle through all his professional and personal development has been about patient care, providing the best and most advanced treatments. Sports is the ultimate eponym for performance. An athlete has to be on stage in front of other people. All other professions can be disguised. Performance, both good and bad, is not always visible. Certainly not in real time. This can breed mediocrity and apathy especially in a healthcare system that at times offers very little incentive to excel. The system promotes volume at the cost of quality. Middlemen in the system grab major profits. They don't often contribute to better patient care.

Dr. Goswami was naturally drawn to sports and athletes. This meant going outside the constraints of mainstream medicine, not an easy route and certainly not the path to riches. One thing never wavered, finding the best treatments for his patients. During multiple sabbaticals over a three-year period, Dr. Goswami traveled, read, learned, and observed natural healing. He realized the potential of one's own stem cells. Much of this process involved unlearning what mainstream medicine had taught him. It was a journey that helped Dr. Goswami not only find the true meaning of healing but also regain his joy in the practice of medicine.

It is unfair for a physician to claim all the credit for successful outcomes. There are some patients who do not do as well. A true physician always learns from patients who have poor outcomes or unexpected complications. Successful patients contribute to their own well-being by taking care of their bodies and focusing on performance. Successful patients fade from memory. The unsuccessful ones stay with the physician for the rest of his life.

The patient author in this book, Kerry Johnson, followed his own journey in the world of professional tennis by battering his body. Living with pain, he continued to play. Fighting pain requires tremendous courage and strength. The wisdom gained through those hard years turned him into a bestselling author and award-winning professional speaker. Writing and speaking at conferences around the world have been his main goals.

After 12 books on a variety of business/motivational topics and 100 speeches a year around the world for four decades, he found a topic he could become even more passionate about. Being in pain is a hard slog. There is no hope. The only objective is to gather enough strength to endure. One report revealed 50% of chronic pain sufferers contemplate suicide. Kerry was one. Stem cell therapy was not only a relief, in many ways it was a salvation. In Kerry's words, "I am now an evangelist of this treatment."

When he sees competitors on the tennis court limping, he asks about their pain. Often these athletes only know of surgery as a last resort. Many can no longer play the sports that brought them enjoyment and emotional release. Kerry now offers a different approach. There is no downside to your own stem cell therapy. It should be the first option before surgery. There are dozens of athletes Kerry wishes he could have counseled before they went under the knife. More than half are worse off as a result of surgery. Their only sin was not knowing about stem cell therapy.

Kerry has become the Billy Graham of the stem cell cure. Wouldn't you be if the only pain relief that has ever worked for you is stem cell intervention? Wouldn't you become a preacher if you could only help that next person get out of pain? How guilty would you feel if you knew how to help a friend but didn't reach out?

Kerry speaks around the world to corporations from Halifax to Hong Kong, from Moscow to Marrakech. His career has been very successful for 40 years. But now there is even more passion. You don't need to accept your injury. You don't need to accept your pain. There is help. Your own cells are the answer. You have hope. The answer lies in your own body's ability to heal. Your own body will heal your pain.

The authors' destinies were bound to intersect. We have shared our knowledge and understanding of stem cells in this book. We have consciously stayed away from medical jargon. The concepts in this book have been oversimplified to make them understandable for the average reader. We assume you have little medical background. Yet you will be able to understand important stem cell concepts.

About this Book

The purpose of this book is to provide you with a basic understanding of the rapidly growing field of stem cell therapy.

- What are the sources of stem cells?
- What are the different types of stem cells?
- How do stem cells work?
- Which stem cells work better for your specific condition?
- What are the differences between foreign stem cells and your own stem cells?
- What are the limitations of stem cells?

As you read this book, you should be able to find answers to these important questions. We also hope the book raises more questions. Only then can medicine truly progress. And ultimately, if you can save some hard-earned money by not falling for a sham "stem cell" treatment, it will be well worth it.

For any treatment to be effective, it is extremely important to understand its scope as well as potential limitations. This book is a culmination of the experience of a physician and several patients. We will attempt to clarify certain concepts, not only about stem cells, but also why we need treatments in the first place. To this end, we have gone beyond the basics of stem cells and addressed concepts that can help you lead a healthy and productive life. We will also discuss the role of nutrition, proper physical conditioning, and injury prevention as well as how to control your emotions and mind. In the end, all healing takes place from within. It's extremely important that we value the precious body nature has given us.

Hopefully the book piques your interest as to the potential of stem cells and their application. The chapters are designed to address conditions for which stem cell therapy may have a potential role. The purpose of patient case histories is to identify and understand their conditions. In order to protect the identity of patients, names have been changed. Several stem cell therapies are emerging, and more data is required to prove their effectiveness.

Each chapter ends with certain key points that can help you decide what's best for you and your family. This book is not a prescription for your condition, neither is it a recommendation for what you should do. Treatment advice should come from a physician who is familiar with your specific condition. Stem cell therapy is a rapidly evolving field involving many different ways (and often claims) of achieving results. Most of these claims unfortunately cannot be truly verified. It is important for you as a potential patient to decipher the vast information. This book will help you cut through the noise so you can make a well-informed decision for you and your loved ones. No single book is comprehensive enough to cover this entire vast topic. We hope through the science and patient experiences shared in this book, you will find the book enlightening and informative as well as entertaining. Ultimately the success of this endeavor lies in patients all over the world making better choices regarding their own health.

Stem cell therapies are extremely new, and with anything new there will be great highs and great lows. This book is ultimately dedicated to the patients who are willing to push the boundaries beyond traditional thinking in an effort to look at better ways of naturally healing themselves.

CHAPTER 1

Welcome to the World of Stem Cells

The entire human body is a collection of cells;
our cells are the fundamental unit of our life.

The Basics

We all start our journey as a single cell. This cell then specializes into different types of cells, which further develop into different organs. As we mature, our cells continue to multiply and replace themselves throughout our lifetime. The basic cells that make all of this possible are called "stem cells."

Stem cells are an integral part of all our organ systems and practically govern our health, disease, and aging. Application of stem cells in the treatment of disease and injury is called "stem cell therapy."

While our knowledge of disease and injury has improved over the past two decades, mainly due to sophisticated imaging techniques, our treatment methods have remained rather primitive.

1

Just as the resolution of your phone screen is dependent on the health of the pixels constituting it, your daily life depends on how well your cells are functioning. How your cells respond to disease and injury determines the symptoms you feel. Unless there is healing at the cell level, you are unlikely to feel better. Medications and surgeries, in most cases, have completely bypassed this scientific truth. While they may have a role to play in certain conditions, we have to focus on healing our bodies by healing our cells.

With this brief understanding, let's answer some commonly asked questions (largely derived from patient consultations) you or your friends and family may have!

1. **What are stem cells?**
    Stem cells are the basic cells that develop and differentiate into different organ cell types. Once our organ systems have matured, stem cells replace old dying cells with new ones throughout the course of our life.

2. **What is the role of stem cells?**
    Cells within every organ of your body have their own life cycle. Stem cells replace those cells. This process is happening 24/7 in your life until your very last moment.

3. **Why are stem cells important?**
    Stem cells make life sustainable. By constantly turning over and replacing old cells with new cells, stem cells make sure our bodies are functioning optimally. They maintain health. When disease or injury strikes your body, your stem cells remove damaged cells and replace them with new cells. This helps your body heal itself and you continue to function.

4. If my body is full of stem cells, why do I need help when I suffer from disease or injury?

Depending on the severity of your condition, your own stem cells may not be able to heal the damage on their own. When the condition is severe and damage is significant, your stem cells need extra help. That extra help so far has been in the form of drugs or surgery.

5. What is stem cell therapy?

If you have a significant disease or injury that your body cannot heal on its own, help is needed. Additional stem cells given to boost your local cells may potentially help you heal. That help (when more stem cells are introduced at the site of disease and injury in an attempt to heal) is called "stem cell therapy."

6. What are the different types of stem cells?

There are many different types of stem cells. Each specialized organ has its own stem cells that help regenerate and repair local cells specific to that organ system. We are still learning about the different populations of stem cells and their functions. The most commonly studied cells are the mesenchymal stem cells found in most of our organ systems. These tend to reside along the blood vessels. Bone marrow, muscle, pancreas, liver, lung, kidney, fat, dental pulp, and joint lining (synovium) are some of the organs rich in mesenchymal stem cells.

7. What are the different sources of stem cells?

There are many different sources of stem cells. The main categories are your own stem cells (autologous) versus stem cells belonging to another individual (foreign). At any stage of your life, you carry your own stem cells. As an adult, your own body carries stem cells in virtually all your organ systems. These stem cells can be harvested from your own body. Stem cells can also be harvested from another person's body at any stage of that person's life. The most common sources are from babies such as embryonic stem cells (pure embryonic stem cells are banned and may involve sacrifice of life). Other sources commercially available are amniotic fluid (fluid surrounding the baby in the mother's womb), the placenta (the site where the baby is attached to the mother in the womb), and the umbilical cord (the cord that attaches the baby to the mother). These are all sources foreign to your body since they belong to another individual. The big concern with foreign stem cells is whether your body will accept or reject them. Their ability to mount an immune reaction and cause other long-term side effects is largely unknown and poorly understood.

8. **I am old; are my stem cells ineffective?**
    There is good news here. Your stem cells do not age at the same rate as your regular cells. Research has shown that a healthy lifestyle can help maintain the potency of your own stem cells. Your own stem cells can be very effective in tissue repair and regeneration despite your age. Studies have shown that we can slow down the aging process by watching the amount of food we eat, doing regular exercise, and managing stress. Having healthy habits makes your own stem cells stronger. This will help if you ever need them. Despite aging, currently your own stem cells are still your best bet when it comes to treatment. Your own cells can be harvested in large numbers, and they can

be delivered fresh back into your body. So both the cell count and the number of live cells from your own source are much higher than most foreign sources can provide.

9. **What conditions can be treated with stem cells?**
    Current stem cell treatments have limited application in athletes and others with sports-related injuries, joint pain, or back pain. Treatments for heart failure, lupus, scleroderma, MS, stroke, macular degeneration, and autism are being offered to selected patients in clinical trials at academic centers. Additional specific stem cells required in conditions such as diabetes, kidney failure, Parkinson's, ALS, lung disease, and several others are in the process of being developed. When it comes to stem cell treatments, "one type does not fit all." Many conditions will require their own types of stem cells and their own treatment protocols. This can get very confusing very quickly. If there is no good mainstream treatment option for your condition, you should explore whether stem cell therapy can benefit you. However, beware of the snake oil salesman. Plenty of clinics advertise and claim they have stem cell treatments for various conditions, but there is no proof that the treatments work.

10. **Are there conditions where stem cells may not be helpful?**
    Even though we would like to think of stem cells as the holy grail of medicine, they have their limitations. At such an early stage of stem cell knowledge, we are still trying to grasp their full potential. Also we have little understanding of their limitations. Our current understanding is that stem cells can help regenerate and repair your damaged cells. They are not going to fundamentally

alter why you suffered from the disease in the first place. Clearly there are certain genetic or congenital conditions in which stem cells may not have a significant role to play. Future treatments such as gene therapy are investigating why some of us are more likely to suffer from a particular condition than others.

11. How are stem cells prepared for treatment?

A lot depends on the source. If they are your own stem cells, they can be harvested or collected from your body by doing a minor procedure. The next step is breaking your tissue down to filter out your own stem cells. They are then ready to be put back into your body. This entire process can be done in the same day at the same sitting. You have the ability to utilize your own fresh stem cells the same day. Alternatively your tissues can be collected and then sent to a laboratory for isolation. Sometimes this involves expansion and or programming of your own stem cells. Your own stem cells are then administered to you at a later date.

Stem cells from foreign sources (those obtained from sources other than your own body) are collected from another individual. This could be from a baby or even another adult. Stem cells acquired from foreign sources require laboratory processing, cleaning, and sometimes expansion and/or programming. Foreign stem cells are frozen in storage until needed for your treatment. Laboratory processing of foreign stem cells should be properly performed in order to minimize the risk of introducing any new disease into your body. Laboratory processing can kill many cells. The steps involved are critical to have enough live cells for an effective treatment.

12. How are my own stem cells collected from my body?

Every part of your body, every organ system, possesses stem cells. You can get your own stem cells from any part of your body. However, the goal is to collect them safely in a way that does not harm your body. Commonly used sites to collect your own stem cells are bone marrow, fat, muscle, tendon, dental pulp, lining of your joints (synovium), skin, and liver. It is hoped that in the near future many more sites will serve as a safe source of collection. Surprisingly, your blood does not contain stem cells. It is a good source of platelets (platelet-rich plasma or PRP) but not stem cells.

13. How are stem cells delivered into my body?

It depends on the intended site of delivery of stem cells, which in turn depends on the condition being treated. Precise delivery of stem cells at the site of disease and injury in your body is critically important in order for you to see results. Stem cells regenerate and repair. Although they secrete valuable growth factors, unless they make it to the site of damage, you are unlikely to see robust results. Currently most stem cells have to be delivered through a targeted injection using very small needles under imaging guidance such as ultrasound or X-rays, videoscope, blood flow, or a direct injection. The important goal is that a sufficient number of live stem cells reach areas where help is needed. Other potential routes such as intravenous, intranasal, intra-arterial, intrathecal (CSF), and inhalational are important to consider. The efficacy and the safety of each one of these routes are still being evaluated in clinical trials.

14. What are the potential risks of stem cell therapy?

Again, it depends upon what kind of stem cells you are getting and how the stem cells are delivered into your body. Your own stem cells carry the least risk. Any manipulation of stem cells in a laboratory or foreign source of stem cells can carry the risk of infection, disease transmission, rejection, and tumor formation. Delivery methods themselves can cause bleeding and additional trauma, although collateral damage is minimal when small needles are used.

15. How many stem cells do I need? Is there a specific number?

Not yet! Unlike the dosage of medications, the exact number of stem cells needed to treat a particular condition in a particular patient is yet unknown. Clearly the greater the extent and severity of damage, the more stem cells that would be needed. No matter what, it would be unreasonable to expect that a single treatment or injection will cure your condition completely. This also depends on how healthy you are otherwise. Several factors may play a role in determining the number of cells and/or number of stem cell treatments you may need.

16. Besides the number of cells, what else is important in a stem cell treatment?

Viability—how many stem cells are alive at the time of your treatment. You can have a high total cell count, but if a significant number of stem cells are dead, you may not see results. This is especially important when a foreign source of stem cells is being used or if the stem cells are being processed in the laboratory. Whenever laboratory processing and cleaning are involved, a certain number of stem cells are bound to be lost. How many live stem cells you get at the time of treatment is important. Another important aspect is the quality of the stem cells. Testing can determine their quality. The hope is that we will also be able to detect any changes in the structure of stem cells and predict how they will behave in your body. The count, quality, and structure of stem cells are all important criteria in minimizing risks and predicting a desired outcome.

17. How many stem cell treatments will I need?

It comes down to what your condition is and how much help your local cells need. For example, an 18-year-old kid playing basketball and suffering his first knee injury is going to heal very differently compared with a 60-year-old skier who has suffered a knee injury and has endured multiple previous knee surgeries. Furthermore, those 60-year-old skiers with similar multiple prior knee injuries and surgeries will heal differently from each other. We are just starting to learn how our cells behave and why patients don't heal the same way. How your stem cell treatment was performed will also determine how many treatments you will need. There are many variables that can affect the efficacy of a stem cell treatment.

18. What is the success rate with stem cell treatment?

This depends on your condition, the source of the stem cells, and the way they are delivered. There are so many different ways of doing stem cell treatments that there can be no apples-to-apples comparison. At least not yet. Due to a lack of standardization, the results are varied. When the treatments are performed correctly for the right reasons, success rates can be around 60% to 70% for joint pain, back pain, and sports injuries. For other conditions, very little is known about how effective the treatments will be. Ongoing research will provide answers in the near future.

19. Why don't some patients see results after stem cell therapy?

No single treatment of any kind is effective in all patients with the same condition. We believe the same is true of stem cell therapy. Our hope is that, in time, as more knowledge is gained, the failures will be minimal. We already know that there is a small group of patients who do not respond to stem cell therapy no matter what. The cause is unknown. But the answer could be genetic in nature.

If all other factors remain the same, outcomes from any procedure depend on three factors:

- Your general health, both physical and mental
- Your environment
- Your genetic makeup

While we don't have much control over the latter, we can do a lot to benefit the first two. Our body's capacity to heal from most conditions is dependent on how healthy we are. With similar conditions, two patients undergoing the same procedure using a physician possessing excellent technical skills can have very different outcomes. Medical treatments aid your body in healing. But ultimate healing takes place from within. No treatment can work unless your body and mind have the ability to heal. With so much emphasis on physical appearance, we have forgotten that the mind controls the body. Thoughts become actions. Our actions in turn determine our life. Everything that makes up the environment we live in, starting with the air we breathe, to the people that surround us, has an impact on our ability to heal.

20. Are stem cell treatments approved by the FDA?

Not yet. With so many different treatments under the "stem cell" umbrella, it has become difficult for any regulation to be formulated. Governments, providers, and commercial suppliers are equally to blame. There is a lack of understanding of the science of stem cells, especially the power of your own stem cells. Some providers manipulate desperate patients. Commercial suppliers are hungry for profits. Many have taken advantage of suffering patients. Many patients are getting fake stem cell treatments or denied a stem cell therapy that could have greatly helped. Either way, many patients end up paying a price. Unfortunately, ignorance and greed often overtake science.

21. Does insurance cover stem cell treatments?

Not yet. Some commercial manufacturers and clinical practices may offer insurance coverage. Generally this is through manipulation of a billing code that may be fraudulent. Unfortunately insurance companies are tied to government regulation. Yet insurance providers have a wonderful opportunity to conduct their own internal studies between patients receiving mainstream treatments and those undergoing recognized forms of stem cell therapy. Isn't the purpose of your health insurance to offer you the best possible treatment?

22. **How much does it cost for stem cell treatment?**

The overall cost depends on the condition that is being treated, the source of the cells being used, and the number of treatments involved. The average cost of a treatment, for example, in a patient with joint pain is between $2,000 and $8,000 per stem cell treatment. We also hear numbers as high as $15,000 to $20,000 per treatment. This wide variation in cost tells us that stem cell therapy is all over the place. There are several ways of doing the treatment. Greed complicates things further. So beware! The lack of standardization makes it difficult to compare results. Further, none of these treatments or protocols have been approved. Published data are sketchy, and robust studies are lacking. We recommend that you look into clinical trials at academic centers. Google should not be your only source when it comes to stem cell treatments!

We hope that these questions and answers satisfied some of your curiosity. And also that you will have even more questions that we can address. That will be the true success of this endeavor. To further your understanding, let's look at some clinical case reports.

CASE STUDY: **NICOLE**

Nicole, a 19-year-old college freshman, was riding on the back of her boyfriend's motorcycle. They were headed to the dorm returning from a late-night party. As they merged onto the freeway, an out-of-control pickup truck hit them. Nicole was ejected into the air, hitting a utility pole. No drugs or alcohol were involved. Nicole became paralyzed from the neck down suffering a severe spinal cord injury. A life brimming with hope came to a halt. A day earlier, she could eat, bathe, dress, text, play, and engage in all the normal activities any other teenager could do. That ended. The psychological and emotional impact on both Nicole and her family was profound. Her younger brother was having a hard time coming to terms with her injury and hospitalization.

Luckily for Nicole, she gained access to a recently developed clinical trial. Stem cells had recently been programmed to grow into nerve cells. They could successfully be implanted into her damaged spinal cord.

Nicole underwent the new treatment. Over the next few weeks, she regained motion in her arms and hands. For the first time in months, she was able to write and even use her phone. This was a huge recovery. Only time will tell whether this was spontaneous. Did she actually benefit from the experimental stem cell therapy, or was it just luck?

Cases like this create faith in the power of stem cells. Although such treatments are now limited to just a handful of patients enrolled in high-powered clinical trials, there is tremendous hope for the future.

CASE STUDY: **SEAN**

Sean was a rising high school football star. He was recruited by a very successful college football program while in 12th grade. He was hoping to eventually transition to the pros. Sean suffered an injury to his knee causing a complete ACL tear with associated meniscal and ligamentous injuries.

It is not uncommon for the knee to suffer extensive damage when an ACL is completely torn. As Sean lay on the field with his leg twisted, his professional career hopes faded. Despite surgical repair and a robust rehab, Sean was unable to play football at the same level. He needed prolonged rest to recover, ruining his chances of landing in the pros. Having a profound love for the game, he now focused his energies on developing younger players. A couple of years out of college, Sean became the head coach at his alma mater high school. He was ecstatic about his new position and looked forward to being a good coach.

Now barely 36, and approximately 17 years after his original surgery, Sean began to notice pain in his treated knee, which progressively became worse. He especially felt discomfort after he ran drills with his players. The pain became persistent. It interfered with his daily life and job. He had always stayed in great shape. There was never any drug or steroid use. But now the pain was unbearable. Since Sean's meniscus was torn and removed at the time of his ACL repair, he did not have much space left between his bones. He would need a knee replacement.

Sean was in the middle of rebuilding his career. Now the thought of undergoing such a major surgery frightened the hell out of him. He had a two-year-old daughter at home. With surgery, there are risks of blood clots, infections, and even future revision surgeries. Sean wanted to save his knee. He shied away from cortisone and gel injections that offered temporary relief. Sean started looking for alternative options. He was able to discover the promise of stem cell therapy. His own stem cells could be drawn from his tissues, and the procedure would be done on the same day at the same sitting.

After his own stem cells were separated, they were injected into his knee. Within the next few weeks, Sean noticed a significant reduction in pain that gradually improved mobility. After the therapy, he was able to get back to his coaching duties without pain meds. He continued to improve. Sean will possibly require additional treatments as time goes by. But he successfully avoided the debilitations of surgery.

These two case histories lay out the current scientific possibilities. However, keep in mind that the term "stem cells" has become a fad. As we noted earlier, it is the latest pitch among snake oil salesmen. It is important to ignore the hype. This craze encompasses a host of treatments, some of which may not even involve true stem cells. The only connection is that they are loosely labeled stem cells. These fad treatments often lead to poor outcomes, unwanted side effects, and complications.

Using fresh stem cells from your own body is a procedure that has been around for more than a decade. It has primarily gained popularity in Europe and Japan. Stem cell treatment is now being performed in some shape or form all over the world. A significant amount of published data have supported many of these treatments. But due to a lack of standardized protocols, these treatment methods have not yet been approved by the FDA and are not currently covered by health insurance. We firmly believe that stem cells will be a major treatment tool in the near future. This book will help separate fact from fiction.

WHAT TO EXPECT

The field of stem cell research is evolving. Different perspectives and ideologies exist. The current lack of standardization further complicates understanding. We hope that the knowledge shared in subsequent chapters will provide a fertile ground to build on. This in turn will help you to make better decisions when seeking stem cell treatment either for yourself or for your loved ones and to become more aware of its potential.

CHAPTER 2

Understanding Disease, Injury, and Aging

First, do no harm.

Breaking It Down

Before we can understand how stem cell therapy works, it is important to know what happens during disease and injury. Now more than ever before, we are starting to look further than just the symptomatic control of conditions. We are trying to identify the root causes. Ideally this should have been done all along with any so-called approved treatments. We are partly to blame, in a society obsessed with fixes that provide immediate satisfaction like fast food. Pharmaceutical companies have thrived on that perception.

Most medications come with serious downsides. Among all the drugs out there, none have done more harm than pain medications. Look at the opioid crisis gripping us all. In the end, we all pay a heavy price directly or indirectly through a ripple effect from this level of immediate gratification.

We are finally investigating what happens in the first place to our cells in disease and injury. How do our cells respond when injury and disease happen? Our hope is that this will point us in the right direction. Some treatments are being developed that are safe and effective and come without much downside.

Stem cell therapy is the latest kid on the block, but it has its own limitations as well. We still need to be careful in developing medications that actually enhance our healing capacity. Surgery should be offered only when its goals and outcomes are well defined. Only then can any treatment be called truly successful. We should all uphold the maxim "First, do no harm." Only then can we maximize our journey and realize our true potential, individually and as a human race.

When a disease or any other medical condition afflicts us, three important things must be first understood:

1. What caused the disease?
2. What is the impact of the disease on local tissues as well as the remainder of the body?
3. How does your body cope with 1 and 2 above?

Let's look at these in further detail.

What Triggers Disease?

The disease triggers in any organ system can be broken down into:

- Trauma and injury related to sports, automobile accidents, and extreme temperatures.

- Congenital defects or genetic predispositions. These are conditions we are born with, such as sickle cell anemia and cerebral palsy, or conditions that we have a tendency toward because of family history, such as heart disease, diabetes, cancer, and certain mental illnesses.
- Environmental influence: pesticides, bacteria, viruses, fungi, alcohol, smoking, drugs, stress.
- Lack of blood flow (arterial blockage) leading to heart attack, stroke.
- Malnutrition, which can cause deficiency (lack of vitamins, protein loss) or excess (obesity, diabetes, high cholesterol).
- Autoimmune responses. The body reacts to its own cells. The most common examples are allergic reactions, rheumatoid arthritis, and lupus.
- Abnormal multiplication of cells due to a variety of factors, some listed above, which results in cancer.
- Aging. As we age, there will be a gradual decline in our ability to renew our cells, although healthy diet and exercise can markedly slow down this decline.

How Disease and Aging Affect Your Cells

Whatever the cause or mechanism of any condition, ultimately it's the local cells that get affected. When the damage is minimal or reversible, we recover. We get some rest and take minor medications, and we are good to go. Natural regeneration and repair occur, and our body is able to replace the mildly damaged cells, thereby restoring our functional capacity. In fact, that's how we all survive the rigors of daily life. But when the damage is significant and/or repetitive, inflammation develops among the local cells within the affected organ. This is due to certain chemicals released from the affected cells and buildup of toxins. The toxins and chemicals also attract pro-inflammatory cells to the affected area. A combination of these sends your local cells into "inflammatory shock." This inflammation does not necessarily mean you see a visible red swollen organ. This inflammation is at the level of your cells. Such inflammation manifesting only at the level of the cells is more sinister and can go undetected for many months to years. Inflammation along with the chemicals released locally by the affected cells causes two main things. One is that it produces symptoms, of which pain is the most common and profound.

Second, inflammation shuts down the local regenerative process through "inflammatory lock." Our own cells become overwhelmed by the damaged cells. Our ability to self-regenerate and repair is markedly decreased. This sets up a vicious cycle of events that lead to further progression of the disease process and injury, which leads to more symptoms and further diminishes our capacity to function. When this process is not addressed in time, it becomes chronic. With the loss of function, the cells lose their ability to replicate. If left untreated, ultimately cell death follows.

Each organ and its cells have different capacities. Depending on what initiated the disease or injury, cell responses may vary. But the underlying theme is inflammation at the cellular level. That is why anti-inflammatories have worked for so long. But now we are starting to understand their side effects and the overall impact on the body. Cortisone and other steroids are very powerful chemicals that suppress inflammation. But their harmful side effects cause weakening of the very cells that are being treated.

An inescapable event is aging. As we age, our cells do slow down a bit. But our ability to regenerate and repair stays strong. Studies have shown that the ability of stem cells to replicate is not impacted as much by aging as are other cells. However, poor diet, lack of exercise, and stress have been shown to suppress the stem cells' ability to function. This not only can impact a cell's capacity to replicate, but also can damage our DNA and shorten chromosomes. This further decreases our cells' ability to replicate and ultimately shortens our life.

Similarly, chronic inflammation anywhere in the body can make our stem cells run out of steam early, impacting not only the quality of our life but also longevity. This highlights how important it is for us to not let any chronic inflammation take root. On the flip side, we can slow down the destruction of our cells and further strengthen our stem cells by watching what we eat, exercising regularly, and managing stress. These three mixed together are the recipe for the best anti-aging cocktail out there!

How the Body Responds to Damage

The body attempts to cope with disease and injury to a certain extent, provided we let it. Rest, proper diet and nutrition, mental clarity, and calmness, along with proper physical exercise, can all help the body heal itself. As inflammation settles down, pain starts to lessen. It is extremely important we let the inflammation subside completely, preventing the condition from progressing to a chronic state.

The body will respond to damage in two ways:

1. When injury or damage is mild, the cells will regenerate.

    Or

2. When the injury or damage is profound, the loss of tissue will result in declining function, and if the decline is extensive, then death will result.

When possible, it is important to focus on regenerative repair and healing by replacing damaged native cells. This process helps us return to optimal function and performance. The rate of tissue regeneration and repair varies in different organs. Bone marrow cells, skin cells, and the lining of our gut replace themselves at a high rate. Organs such as the kidneys, liver, and lungs repair at a much slower pace. Tissues such as brain cells (neurons) or heart cardiac muscle cells do not regenerate on their own. Injuries in these organs generally end up in scar tissue formation with loss of function.

CASE STUDY: **REZA**

Reza, a 32-year-old software programmer, started feeling cramping abdominal pain accompanied by loose stools about six years ago. At the time he was a sales manager for a reputable pharmaceutical company. His erratic bowel movements interfered with his job. He was always on the lookout for a nearby restroom. He inconveniently had to plan ahead on most of his sales trips. He tried some dietary modifications, but the symptoms persisted. He also noticed some blood-stained stools. After a colonoscopy and biopsy, he was diagnosed with ulcerative colitis.

With medications, Reza would feel good for a few months. But his symptoms would return with a vengeance. He eventually had to give up his sales career and retrained as a software programmer in an effort to work from home. He became physically, psychologically, and socially devastated. Last year, reluctantly, he agreed to undergo colectomy surgery in which nearly his entire colon was removed. He has some relief now but has to deal with the side effects of such a major surgery.

Along with Crohn's disease, ulcerative colitis is part of the spectrum of inflammatory bowel disease that affects about 2 million people in North America. And the incidence of these maladies is rising in many developing countries. In this disease, the lining of the bowel is inflamed and starts destroying local cells. The exact cause is unknown. But family history, immune reaction, and environmental bacteria or toxins can play a role.

Inflammation, the Secret Killer

We need to play close attention to the role inflammation plays. Inflammation is an attempt by our body to control disease and injury. Left unchecked, inflammation can damage cells and create a toxic environment. Inflammation can affect local tissue and cells impacted by disease and injury. But it also has a systemic effect on the rest of the body. One common example is fever caused by inflammation anywhere in the body. The consequences can be devastating. Significant injuries and chronic conditions overwhelm the body and need help in order to get things under control. Medications and surgery have been our primary options so far. However, these approaches do not necessarily address the root cause of what's happening at the cellular level. Even when effective, they cause negative side effects and collateral damage. Surgery along with subsequent immobilization can induce more inflammation.

CASE STUDY: **PHILIP**

Philip is a 50-year-old who has been an insurance company administrator for 25 years. Over the last 12 months, both his knees have been hurting. When he wakes up in the morning, his joints stiffen up. He feels stiffness and pain even when rising from his desk. Some days the pain can be pretty severe. Philip has resorted to over-the-counter pain medications.

Philip decided to go see his doctor to find out what led to his knee pain. There has been no recent injury or trauma. He has led a pretty regular life. His wife has worked at an administrative job at a local hospital for the past 20 years. They have a son now 22, just out of college. Philip is moderately built with a body mass index of about 27. He doesn't remember ever having a problem with his knees before. Both Philip's parents have age-related aches and pains consistent with osteoarthritis.

So why do our joints hurt as we age? Especially when there have been no specific injuries? We have always thought that joint pain was due to wear and tear. But research has recently shown that there might be more happening inside the joint contributing to pain. It is more than simply wear and tear.

We are starting to understand what happens at the cellular level. It could be a combination of things. A sedentary lifestyle, aging, and a genetic predisposition (a family history) can all contribute to joint pain and the early onset of osteoarthritis. As we age, the cells within cartilage go into a state of inflammation, altering their ability to heal. The inflammation also alters the ability of joints to handle weight and pressure. A genetic predisposition to osteoarthritis can speed up this process. Even during youth, declining activity and a sedentary lifestyle cause muscles to go weak. The muscles are unable to support the joint. These events together set up a chain reaction. One thing leads to another, and soon pain starts to become part of our life. The good news is that we can slow down this process.

Since injury or disease disturbs our cells, all repair and healing also has to occur at the level of our cells. Stem cell treatments are based on the concept of replacing these damaged cells with new cells, leading to tissue growth. The new cells help repair diseased or injured tissues. As well, stem cells are known to have a powerful anti-inflammatory effect. In certain scenarios stem cells can help fight inflammation at the cellular level and preserve natural tissue without much downside. As stem cell treatments develop, they will have to be tailored to the particular tissues or cell types they are attempting to regenerate. They can also alter our immune environment. This further helps to clean up the toxic inflammatory environment and thus promote healing. Preliminary research is showing promise, and the hope is that a cure for many conditions is in the near future.

Factors That Impact Healing

No matter what the treatment, there are certain elements within our environment and body that can actually interfere with the healing process. Your goal should be to minimize the impact on your body's ability to heal. Factors both inside you and outside in your environment may have to be controlled for optimal healing.

One important thing to do after any procedure or treatment is to reduce local pressure or force. It is important to rest the part that has been treated. As tissue regeneration and repair takes place, you should prevent the healing cells from pulling apart or becoming disrupted. You want the healing cells to line up. A lack of rest can only lead to distortion and suboptimal healing.

Next it is important that your nutrition is good. A deficiency of certain proteins, vitamins, and minerals (especially vitamin C) can interfere with cell multiplication and regeneration. This can delay the healing process and/or result in the development of weaker tissues.

Both infection and diabetes can compromise the regenerative capacity of your cells and interfere with healing. And not only can they result in improper healing, but diabetes and infection can create severe complications affecting the whole body.

Maintaining good circulation and blood flow where the healing is taking place is critically important for tissues to heal. If you do not have good circulation, even good nutrition may not reach the body part where help is needed. Staying well hydrated is a simple way of making sure you have good circulation. Obviously, watching what you eat and keeping your cholesterol under control can only improve blood flow. Your cells (including stem cells) need to stay in a state of good hydration for important cellular functions to take place.

Managing Stress

Mental stress, self-doubt, and negative thinking all suppress the natural ability of our bodies to fight disease. This is the X factor that is generally not addressed in mainstream medicine. Patients don't acknowledge it, and most physicians are not equipped to handle it. The mind is a powerful tool. When used correctly, it can help us fight great odds. When not used well, it can create havoc. The body follows the mind.

The above factors impact our ability to heal no matter what treatment we undergo. This is true with medications, surgeries, and even stem cell treatments. If you are really looking for results, pay attention to fundamentals.

CASE STUDY: RON

Ron was proud of his 20 years as a special-needs teacher. Now 48, he was in the same school district he started in. Ron had several opportunities to move up the administrative ranks. But he loved the kids. He always enjoyed a good joke, and his students loved him for it. Special education can be high stress. But Ron had a positive outlook. Ron was brought up in a family with plenty of love and abundance. Helping those in need brought him great pleasure.

Ron was hooked on sodas and Twinkies. He would have a Big Gulp cup in his hand as he walked through the corridors. Life progressed, and his habits stayed the same. One evening Ron started having persistent chest pains. He had to be hospitalized. After angiography, a blockage in one of his arteries was identified. A metal stent was placed to open up his artery. Ron had a body mass index of 38 and was diagnosed with obesity. But the additional and more severe diagnosis was type 2 diabetes. Inflammatory markers in his blood work were elevated. Ron also had suffered from severe constipation for several years. Ron was started on a long list of medications. He was disappointed in himself for not taking care of his health. When Ron got out of the hospital, he was determined to change his life and be an example for the students.

Obesity and inflammation are two sides of the same coin. Obesity can lead to inflammation, and inflammation can lead to obesity. We now understand more about what happens to the cells in diabetic patients. Inflammation due to diabetes is widespread throughout the body. It can affect many organs at the same time. Inflammation unfortunately interferes with stem cells and their ability to regenerate and repair. Inflammation then starts affecting the function of normal cells. Left unchecked, inflammation can cause strokes, renal failure, and nonhealing wounds.

What starts inflammation in the first place is unclear. While a genetic predisposition to obesity is known, not much can be done about it. Several other theories exist, especially one involving the gut microbes, the bacteria in your bowel. As mentioned above, Ron had been severely constipated for several years. It could be a combination of factors. Poor diet and lack of exercise are prime examples. It is extremely important that diabetics follow a regimen of weight loss, caloric restriction, and regular exercise to keep their diabetes under control. Staying hydrated every day and eating pomegranates can help reduce inflammation of the cells in diabetes.

We hope that by now you have a better understanding of what happens when you are not feeling well. Think about what your cells are undergoing and how inflammation affects them. Address the root cause and not just the symptoms. Do everything in your power to make your cells healthy again. Only then is your healing complete. Next we will look at how stem cells may help you in your efforts to heal naturally.

KEY TAKEAWAYS

1. Disease and injury lead to inflammation.
2. Inflammation of the cells stops regeneration and repair.
3. Stem cells are extremely potent anti-inflammatories.
4. Fresh food + exercise + positive mindset = best anti-aging cocktail.

CHAPTER 3

How Stem Cells Work

We are powered by our stem cells from conception to death.

Understanding Fundamentals

Wonder how many people would get a haircut if our hair could not regrow! That cut on your finger—a surgeon can stitch it up to bring the skin edges together, but ultimately the skin closes up because of cell growth and multiplication. Though we may not be aware of it at all times, cell multiplication and replacement is a fundamental process that goes on in our body 24/7. Unfortunately, the dreaded disease cancer only exists because our cells replicate. Cancer is just a manifestation of the regeneration and replication process gone awry! There happen to be too many cells in one place; cell multiplication is out of control. In most cases, a pathologist can only determine cancer when the cells are compared with an area of normal cells. Cancer cells actually look like their own host cells.

Stem Cells Can Form Other Cells

Let's expand further by exploring this question: What is a stem cell? And the answer is that a stem cell is a cell capable of self-renewal and capable of forming other cells. We all start our journey as a stem cell. The self-renewal capability of your stem cells is maintained throughout your life. It is the ability to grow into other cells that varies at different stages of your life. At the embryonic stage, the stem cell is capable of growing into any kind of cell or organ system. As you mature, your stem cells are able to grow only into cells they are surrounded by. This is what unfolds in their natural state. Of course, a stem cell can be programmed in a laboratory to grow into a particular type of cell. The process involved in reprogramming a stem cell is currently an area of tremendous research. Also, different tissues have different regenerative capacity. That means different stem cells behave differently. Within the world of stem cells, there are different types. Various stem cells may be required depending on the particular condition being treated. A stem cell that heals your knee will not cure your diabetes! Stem cell treatments are most effective when they replace or repair cells that are missing. So when the cartilage in your joint is worn out, you need stem cells that are capable of regenerating the cartilage. When you have diabetes due to lack of insulin production, you will need stem cells that are capable of producing insulin.

In the past, healing has been largely dominated by chemicals that can suppress the symptoms of pain. Anti-inflammatories such as NSAIDs and steroids have been commonly used. Drugs that are designed to suppress the inflammation end up suppressing the function of those very same cells that are in need of healing, causing further harm. Our symptoms may resolve in the short run, but at the same time, these medications can be very toxic. These medications interfere with cell function rather than promote regeneration and repair. There is a reason why most medications stop working after a while; the cells become so damaged they become resistant.

As we have learned, the presence of inflammation takes away the ability of your cells to multiply and replace themselves. That is why inflammation is the basis of most conditions that take root in your body. This inflammatory state then diminishes the ability of the local cells to perform any meaningful repair or healing. Common conditions such as joint pain, tendinitis, asthma, arterial blockage, and hepatitis are all examples of chronic inflammation. Uncontrolled inflammation is the root cause of many conditions that afflict us.

Your Body Naturally Heals Itself

Your body naturally heals itself daily. When you sprain an ankle or suffer a minor injury, repair and regeneration sets in, and you heal. That is how you survive. Your body fixes minor issues and renews cells. But when the injury is more profound or repetitive, the local cells are not able to perform continued meaningful repair or regeneration. For example, let's take tennis elbow. This is an initial sprain or inflammation at the site of the muscle attaching to the elbow bone. When that early inflammation does not get a chance to heal, the inflammatory process becomes chronic. Slowly it gets to a stage that will require some form of treatment to get relief. Sometimes we make the process worse by not resting. This is seen very commonly among athletes. Without providing rest to the body part that's hurting, inflammation persists and can become chronic.

Regenerative treatment is the basic fundamental concept that aims to jump-start your local cells to help repair cell damage. And, of course, as you know by now, one major tool in the box of regenerative treatments is stem cells. The single most important property of stem cells is that they can exert a strong anti-inflammatory effect. Stem cells can clean up inflammation at the cellular level without causing any side effects. This is contrary to what you have experienced with NSAIDs and steroids. Stem cells exert a major impact on healing by not only growing new cells, but also secreting certain growth compounds that make the local environment at the site of injury healthy. That allows new cells to form and start functioning normally. This is how regeneration and repair happens and you ultimately heal. Nature's best gift to us!

Five Important Stem Cell Functions

Besides being powerful anti-inflammatories, stem cells perform many functions that aid in regeneration and repair. There are five important functions a stem cell performs. These five main actions are how stem cells help you in fighting injury and disease:

1. They replace dead cells by forming new cells.
2. They release growth factors and compounds that promote cell growth.
3. They promote blood flow in the area of healing by forming tiny new blood vessels.
4. They cancel out the body's own inflammatory responses.
5. They slow the breakdown process.

All of the above mechanisms lead to a healthy local environment among the cells. An environment that is more conducive to repair and regeneration.

These functions are critical to the efficacy and effectiveness of stem cells. They help define the possible applications of stem cells and the role they can play in a variety of conditions. Often stem cells are thought of as something that will create a whole new joint, organ, or even a duplicate copy of your body. And someday we may get there. For now the stem cells' most important job is regeneration and repair. The stem cells work in conjunction with your local cells to help remove inflammation and promote blood flow. This will allow nutrients to reach the problem area, further aiding the healing process. Better blood flow helps remove toxic waste material and reduce inflammation. In essence, stem cells work to improve the local environment at the site of injury and disease. A healthier environment then jump-starts the local cells to function again.

In order for stem cells to do their job, they need to be delivered precisely to the site of disease or injury. Unless stem cells reach that site, they cannot modify the local environment of the damaged cells. Stem cells continue to multiply and replicate and repair the cells as time goes along. However, we do not have the full capability to do this for every condition. A more realistic application of stem cells for now is in the area of joint pain and sports injury. Stem cells have provided a much-needed alternative for the management of joint pain, tendinitis, plantar fasciitis, back pain, and sports injuries.

CASE STUDY: **SAMIR**

Samir, a 40-year-old pharmacist, has complained of pain in his feet for years. He has been diagnosed with plantar fasciitis. His profession requires standing for long hours and certainly has contributed to his condition. Samir has tried physical therapy, has had cortisone injections multiple times, and has sought opinions from numerous doctors. Except for a few days of intermittent relief, his pain has always been there. Samir has been told by several doctors that he just has to learn to live with the condition. There may not be any cure.

Samir's older brother is a primary care physician in the community and knew of a doctor who specialized in stem cell treatments. He referred Samir to his physician friend. Samir was evaluated. Using ultrasound and X-rays for guidance, the doctor gave Samir a single treatment of Samir's own stem cells. The injections were made at multiple sites within the plantar fascia. Samir noticed a 50% reduction in his pain two weeks after treatment. He was assessed in follow-up and received one more treatment to the plantar fascia. Samir has been pain-free for the past two years.

CASE STUDY: **ALBERT AND HIS MOTHER**

Albert has been taking care of his mother, who has suffered from Parkinson's disease for several years. He's hired the best caregivers to help his mom deal with this disabling condition. She's had numerous treatments over the years that have seemed to help her. But she still cannot function independently and needs help with daily activities. Between work and taking care of his mother, Albert has very little time for anything else. He's completely dedicated to making sure that he can do the best for his mother.

Recently Albert noticed a lot of stem cell advertisements targeting people with Parkinson's disease. He was curious. During the next visit to his mother's doctor, Albert inquired about the role of stem cells for her.

Parkinson's is a condition where there is a loss of dopamine-producing brain cells. Dopamine helps brain cells communicate with each other. The lack of dopamine leads to miscommunication among the brain cells that affect the patient's movement. As you can imagine, stem cells in Parkinson's should have the ability to grow new cells to replace the ones that were lost. But as we noted earlier in the book, brain cells do not regenerate readily. The use of stem cells in Parkinson's is a sophisticated process and will have to be studied in a laboratory. After the right stem cells are found, those stem cells will have to be delivered into the specific area of the brain affected in Parkinson's. One can imagine how complex and risky that procedure could be. There is also the possibility of negative side effects and complications that we may not be aware of. So even though some clinics advertise using stem cells from the patient's fat or bone marrow or from a newborn baby's umbilical cord, these cells do not have the sophistication to grow into brain cells. These cells are administered intravenously and never make it to the area of the brain affected in Parkinson's. This is a total waste of time and money along with unknown risks.

Still, it is important to know that there is significant ongoing research with stem cells especially derived from an embryonic stage or manufactured stem cells, either of which can then be programmed to grow into the brain cells needed for Parkinson's disease. This research is at its very early stages. You should inquire about clinical trials conducted at academic centers. This at least will assure that you are getting the right stem cell treatment. You can also make sure the risks and side effects are being adequately monitored.

It is understandable why patients and their families feel the desperate need to ease the suffering of their loved ones. We are often willing and tempted to buy into the hype of stem cells. Unfortunately, this only takes away valuable resources that can be used to improve the patient's quality of life.

One Size Doesn't Fit All

When it comes to stem cell therapy, one size does not fit all! A stem cell treatment that can alleviate your joint pain will not cure your blindness, your child's autism, or your grandpa's Alzheimer's! It is appalling how commercial clinics oversell the ability of stem cells to be a cure for a myriad of conditions. Unfortunately, this creates public mistrust and brings on the wrath of regulatory agencies.

Unless cells grow, stem cell therapy will not be effective. How embryonic stem cells are collected, how umbilical cord blood is collected, and how your own tissues are collected can involve different levels of complexity. How stem cells are gleaned or isolated from their sources has a major impact on your treatment. For example, when your own fat or bone marrow is collected, how is it broken down to get a concentrate of your own adult stem cells? Merely putting fat back into the joint is not stem cell therapy! Two patients getting stem cell treatment for a painful joint, using their own fat stem cells, can end up getting two entirely different treatments. In one, the fat will be injected without being broken down. In the other, the fat will be broken down. Your own stem cells will be isolated and then injected into your joint. An important point to understand is that fat contains many different cells, including stem cells. Fat cells are not stem cells. Therefore, it is very important to break down the fat in order to isolate your stem cells, discarding the remainder of unwanted fat cells. Fat is merely acting as an easily available source of your stem cells. Once you have a concentrate of stem cells ready, the next step is to deliver them to the area needing help. How will this be done? Are the cells getting into the joint space? Are they getting to the area of inflammation? Some clinics give intravenous (IV) injections of stem cells. The majority of stem cells given intravenously can get filtered in the lung. It depends on the condition being treated. But don't expect an intravenous injection of stem cells to heal your knee joint. Unless the cells reach the area of damage, they won't be effective. Similarly, cells for conditions affecting the brain may have to be implanted directly into the damaged part of the brain. Research is being conducted to answer some of the questions. Delivery routes and methods for different clinical conditions will vary and have to be clearly established. Until then, we may not be able to predict outcomes or compare results. Unfortunately, there is no apples-to-apples comparison among stem cell treatments yet!

CASE STUDY: **MR. KAPOOR AND HIS DAUGHTER PRIYA**

Mr. Kapoor is a 65-year-old real estate magnate who has traveled the world and loves to golf. He has played at some of the best-known international courses and even carries his own clubs. About seven years ago, his right shoulder started to hurt after playing. It progressively got worse. He was unable to lie on his right side. Shoulder pain kept him up most nights. He had an MRI evaluation that showed a significant, but not complete, rotator cuff tear. He wanted to avoid surgery or any other toxic medications or injections. He started exploring alternatives. After doing thorough research and getting opinions at three different stem cell clinics, Mr. Kapoor underwent stem cell treatment. He received an injection of his own stem cells harvested from his fat and bone marrow. His recovery was uneventful. Over the next two months he gradually resumed playing.

About two years ago, his 21-year-old daughter Priya was diagnosed with type 1 diabetes. Diabetes and its treatment take not only a physical toll, but a psychological one as well. This diagnosis impacts not only the patient but close family members. Determined to find a better cure for his daughter, and given that Mr. Kapoor had such a good experience with stem cells for his shoulder, he contacted the clinic he had gone to, inquiring about stem cell treatment for diabetes. He was told that his daughter could undergo a similar stem cell procedure like the one for his shoulder. The cells would be administered intravenously. Mr. Kapoor was quoted a price that was three times the cost he paid for his shoulder treatment. Mr. Kapoor trusted the clinic and took his daughter for the treatments. He was also advised that she could stop her insulin since the stem cell treatment would cure her diabetes.

Ms. Priya Kapoor received three treatments over three months. There was no improvement in her blood sugar level. The Kapoors were advised to pay for more treatments. In the meantime, Priya started having dizzy spells, and her vision became fuzzy. She also developed tingling and numbness in her feet. One day out of the blue, she noted an ulcer on her little toe. Over the next two weeks, the toe turned black; it was then Mr. Kapoor got alarmed and rushed Priya to a local hospital. The diagnosis was diabetic ulcer with gangrene of the toe. The dead toe had to be amputated. Tests showed that Priya had sky-high blood sugar levels. Her A1C was 14 (normally between 4 and 5.6) and she was heading into major complications due to uncontrolled diabetes. She had stopped taking her insulin on the advice of the stem cell clinic.

Mr. Kapoor had shown blind faith in the physicians. This highlights the dilemma you're likely to face. On one hand, your own stem cells are capable of regenerating tissue like bones, joints, muscles, and cartilage. However, the same cells are not going to increase the production of insulin. They are not going to regenerate and repair diabetes. You need insulin from the outside to control your blood sugar level. Uncontrolled high blood sugar levels can lead to deadly complications, which Priya had started to experience. That is the level of complexity we need to understand.

The questions that need to be answered are: What stems cells are necessary for what condition, and how will they be administered? Cells given through a regular IV are probably not going to be effective. Most cells get filtered in the lung. Don't expect those trapped cells in the lungs to regenerate and repair your pancreas to start making more insulin. This is not a treatment for diabetes, and these are not the stem cells for treatment of diabetes.

Great research is being conducted using embryonic and programmed stem cells that are capable of regenerating insulin-producing cells. Those stem cells can be directly implanted into your body either in the pancreas or at a location where new insulin-producing cells can grow. Again, not all stem cell treatments are the same. They may sound the same in terms of their title, so be careful!

KEY TAKEAWAYS

1. Not all stem cell treatments are the same. The source of the stem cells and the way they are processed prior to you getting them are both critical to the outcome.
2. Different conditions will need different types of stem cells. Your arthritis will not respond to the same stem cells as your diabetes will.
3. In order to be effective, live stem cells must reach the area of damage in your body where help is needed.
4. Multiple stem cell treatments may be required, depending on the nature and extent of your condition.
5. Just like any other treatment, stem cell treatments are most effective when you take care of your body and maintain good general health.

CHAPTER 4

Sources and Types of Stem Cells

The good, the bad, and the ugly.

Stem Cells Help Grow New Cells

If stem cell treatments are properly developed, they have the potential to become as revolutionary as the discovery of penicillin. Just as antibiotics have saved many lives, stem cell treatments can also save many patients who have hit a dead end with mainstream medicine.

When disease or injury happens, there is cell damage. When significant disease or injury happens, cell death can ensue. As we have learned in previous chapters, a variety of toxins and inflammatory compounds are released by damaged or dying cells. These toxins take away the ability of your local stem cells to regenerate. You develop symptoms, and your ability to perform decreases. In order to get the local stem cells functioning again, additional stem cells are needed. This forms the basis of stem cell therapy.

The stem cells help replace damaged and dying cells with new cells that are healthy and functional. Stem cells are also powerful anti-inflammatories and help resolve the local inflammation by neutralizing toxins. This improves the local environment of the cells. The tissue regeneration and growth process then takes place. But one fact we must all agree on is that stem cell treatment can only work if the particular damaged cells are replaced. That means that stem cell treatment must be tailored to your specific condition; otherwise you are unlikely to see any significant benefits.

Unscrupulous Clinics

We begin this section with the tale of Mr. Patel.

CASE STUDY: **MR. PATEL**

Mr. Patel, a 57-year-old businessman in the hospitality industry, started developing knee pain. Initially he used some natural remedies to quell the pain and in general ignored it. Mr. Patel had taken good care of his body with no past injuries. Soon, though, the pain started to interfere with golf. Enjoying a chilled beer after a round of golf with his dear friends on Sundays was his only respite from a stressful career, and so he looked for a new solution. Mr. Patel saw an ad in a local newspaper about stem cell treatments for knee pain. He had already heard of stem cells and their potential, and so he made an appointment for an evaluation. He was seen by a physician and was told his knees were very bad and he would soon need replacement surgery. This physician did not perform any imaging, but instead played upon Mr. Patel's fears to scare him into signing up for stem cell therapy without confirming the diagnosis. Mr. Patel was told that one injection of stem cells should make his knees healthy for the rest of his life. He was told he would be getting fresh baby cells delivered through an IV. Mr. Patel was also told there would be no risks. He asked about using his own cells and was told they were too old to provide any benefit. Seeing no other viable option to avoid surgery, Mr. Patel signed up.

He arrived at the clinic one morning, and an IV was placed in his arm. Then the so-called stem cells were injected through an IV. Mr. Patel got no written notification about the exact nature of the cells, or their count, or their viability. Three months after the procedure, Mr. Patel's knee pain worsened. During a follow-up visit, he was told the treatment did not work for him because his body was too far gone.

Despondent, Mr. Patel started seeking opinions from other doctors. This time he got an ultrasound, X-rays, and MRI imaging. He had a moderate degree of degeneration but still plenty of joint space. Mr. Patel was nowhere near needing joint replacement surgery. He was offered a cortisone or hyaluronic acid injection, which he refused. He sought the opinion of a physician specializing in regenerative medicine. After, he received an injection of PRP (platelet-rich plasma). This reduced the inflammation in his knee joint. He was back playing golf. PRP, derived from his own blood, with his own cells, avoided any side effects and prevented further damage to his own tissues.

While there were several red flags in Mr. Patel's case, it is not uncommon for people to fall prey to clinics promoting stem cell methodologies with no scientific basis. Let's take a look at another patient.

CASE STUDY: **THE OPHTHALMOLOGIST**

Dr. Nina, a practicing ophthalmologist specializing in eye surgery, had damage to one of her knees from years of standing. She was in her early 60s. She had read and researched a little bit about stem cell treatments. Obviously, she was not ready to go under the knife and get a total knee replacement, although this was recommended. She also had a little bit more understanding than the normal layperson about foreign stem cells and associated risks. She also knew that intravenously delivered cells have no role to play. They would be filtered by her lungs and unable to reach her knee.

The eye doctor opted for her own fat-derived stem cells. Approximately 40 mL of fat was aspirated and squished around between two syringes and injected into her knee. That night she was in severe pain. By the next morning, her knee had swelled up. She was told she had an inflammatory reaction. One year after, this busy professional was still reeling with knee pain. She had very few good but mostly bad days. What really went wrong here?

One day, one of her own patients spoke about his entirely different experience with knee stem cell treatment. This gentleman was in so much pain that he walked with a cane. A few months after his own stem cell treatment, he was walking on his own and becoming more and more active. His treatment was done at a clinic that specializes in regenerative medicine and stem cell treatments. His own blood, bone marrow, and fat were used as sources for isolating his stem cells. The treatments were done over three sittings, three to six months apart. All cells were injected into his damaged knee under X-ray imaging guidance. His physician demonstrated that the flow of cells around the joint was critical in ensuring all damaged and worn-out areas would heal. His only side effect was losing an inch around his waist! He didn't remember how much fat was removed. But it certainly was not a mere 40 cc.

As you can see, these cases highlight how many patients fall into a trap. On the surface, treatments labeled "stem cell" can mean nothing. Mr. Patel received cells intravenously that likely never made it to his knee joint. Given the foreign source of the cells, there were never enough to begin with.

The second patient, the ophthalmologist, realized the safety and potential of her own stem cells. Her procedure was just not performed in the right manner. Fat has no place in a joint. Fat is pro-inflammatory. The oil inside fat can cause serious damage and may even calcify (become solid). In the long run, this could make your condition worse.

When people say their bone marrow or fat is being used to treat their joint pain, it means that bone marrow or fat is being used as a source to collect their own stem cells. It is not the bone marrow or fat itself that's going into the joint. What should be injected into your joint should be only your own stem cells. At least that's how the treatment needs to be done; otherwise you're not going to see results, and complications can develop. The quantity of fat harvested was also too low. How much is enough? An exact number is not known; it depends on the patient, his or her condition, and the extent of damage that needs to be repaired. Once fat is broken down, there should be enough stem cells left to do the repair. Harvesting just a little fat makes no sense.

The Spectrum

Before we talk about stem cell treatments, it's important for you to understand the kinds of stem cells that are available. "Stem cell" as a term tells you nothing. It has different meanings for different people. The previous patient case histories highlight how important it is that you understand the stem cells you are getting! What role do stem cells play in your condition? How will the treatment be performed? What will be your follow-up? What results can you expect?

In the universe of stem cell therapies, there are a myriad of different treatments, all labeled the same! So many therapies and so many different sources of cells. It becomes hard to sort through the maze. Which are effective and which are good, bad, or ugly can become murky. We will review the spectrum of stem cells available mostly in terms of their sources. Different types of stem cells grow specific tissue. This area is in its infancy, and a lot more research is needed. Finally, no matter the source or type of stem cells, how many live stem cells are delivered to the area of damage is a critical element of the treatment. The hope is that this review will help you stay away from the snake oil salesman!

Stem cells can be derived from foreign sources or from your own body. Foreign or external sources—stem cells from another individual—include:

- Embryonic stem cells (ESCs), which are restricted to research only. Commercial use is illegal.
- Amniotic fluid/membrane (fluid surrounding the baby in the womb).
- Placenta (the site where the fetus attaches to the mother via the umbilical cord).
- Umbilical cord (the conduit through which nutrition is supplied to the fetus and waste is removed). There are two types:
    a. Wharton's jelly stem cells (supportive tissue within the umbilical cord)

> b. Umbilical cord blood cells (collected from blood vessels within the umbilical cord)

- Donor adult stem cells, which are stem cells collected from another adult and then programmed or modified in the laboratory.

Your own stem cells are called "autologous." These stem cells are collected from your own body and reinjected into your body. Common collection sites are your blood, bone marrow, fat (adipose tissue), muscle, tendon, dental pulp, synovium (lining of the joint), cartilage, skin, liver, and stored cord blood.

Now let's discuss each of these two types of sources in detail.

Foreign Stem Cell Sources

As noted above, foreign or external sources are sources other than your own body. The stem cells from these sources are also sometimes classified as "allogenic."

Embryonic stem cells—these are how we all started our journey—were once considered the holy grail of medicine. But pure embryonic stem cells have been banned because of the sacrifice of human life involved. They certainly have the potential to grow into any kind of cells. However, moral, ethical, and now scientific constraints limit their use. In fact, they have been shown to be potentially dangerous. A cell with someone else's DNA will need to be heavily programmed to help another individual. Also, over the past two decades, significant research in the field of adult stem cells has shown great promise in the reprogramming of your own mature cells.

Other foreign sources belonging to newborn babies, such as amniotic, placental, or umbilical cord, clearly don't require a sacrifice of life. Their commercial supply is growing. These sources can be collected during or after pregnancy without harm to the fetus or the baby. There are a growing number of companies producing a variety of amniotic, placental, Wharton's jelly, and cord cell products. All require that the donor be evaluated for any transmissible disease. The donor sample needs to be tested for infection. After testing, the cells are frozen until ready for use. However, due to post-collection processing and freezing, the actual number of live stem cells found in these sources can vary a lot. And so do the clinical benefits.

Almost all foreign sources require some kind of laboratory processing in order to clean and sterilize the cells. These cells can be stored, packaged, and delivered in frozen containers. The problem is that the methods involved in the processing of foreign cells aren't standardized. Some products offer dry powdered stem cells. In all likelihood, the cells are dead by the time you receive them. Furthermore, risk of disease transmission or infection or even biological alteration cannot be entirely ruled out. Any amount of donor screening, testing, and sterilization does not guarantee that a foreign disease won't be transferred into your body.

Another area of uncertainty is rejection by your body of these foreign stem cells. The argument that a newborn baby has immature cells not capable of mounting a reaction in your body has no scientific basis. A newborn baby is about nine months old at the time of birth. Though the newborn is certainly less mature than an adult, a reaction or rejection cannot be ruled out. Also, although reaction or rejection of a foreign substance does not necessarily occur on first exposure, repeated injections can mount a negative response within your body.

In terms of their collection, foreign cells do not require the harvesting of your tissues. You do not have to undergo any harvesting procedure other than getting the cell injection. Sometimes foreign stem cells are sold with the premise that they are more potent than your own stem cells. The concern is that your own cells may be weaker due to aging. This is not necessarily true, and several scientific studies have shown that your own stem cells maintain potency despite aging.

Irrespective of the source, several variables such as cell count, viability, methods, and routes of injecting the cells into your body determine outcomes. Additionally, the nature of your condition and how your stem cell treatment is performed impact the outcome you are seeking.

Your Own Stem Cells (Autologous)

While foreign sources can provide some stem cells, the largest source is your own body! Right off the bat. No risk of disease transmission and no rejection! Let's dig deeper.

Right now, there are two main sources of autologous cells that can be used to regenerate your body. The two commonly used tissues as sources are your bone marrow and your fat. Cells can be harvested and isolated from these tissues and then injected back into your body in a same-day, same-sitting procedure. You will have to undergo a harvesting procedure where these sources are collected.

The techniques for collecting bone marrow and fat are well defined. We have been safely doing bone marrow collection as well as liposuction for years. Although slightly different when the goal is to recover stem cells, the techniques are refined and extremely safe in experienced hands. There is no downside or discomfort with any of the harvesting.

There are a few other source tissues currently being studied including muscle, synovium, dental pulp, skin, and liver. Greater understanding of the techniques involved for these tissues is needed. One important distinction here is this: Peripheral blood does not contain stem cells. This means that blood-based treatments as the sole treatment, such as PRP (which is excellent in controlling inflammation), lack regenerative capacity.

Stem cells are present in each organ system. That's how your body heals and repairs on a daily basis. The question is, How much bone marrow and how much fat need to be collected? And how are your stem cells isolated from these sources? Merely putting blood, bone marrow, or fat into a joint does not represent stem cell therapy. In fact, such misguided ventures can be counterproductive.

Given so many variables involved, it is hard to do an apples-to-apples comparison of each procedure to figure out what kind of treatment will be most effective. Robust scientific studies are urgently needed to answer some of the questions raised here. The application of your own stem cells has shown some preliminary benefits especially in the area of orthopedics and sports medicine. Some unsubstantiated claims are being made for certain other conditions like MS, Parkinson's, autism, and Alzheimer's. However, these conditions will require a markedly different approach than that used for treating someone's painful joint. Different stem cell types, a high number of cells, innovative methods of delivering them, and multiple treatments may be required. Some well-designed research programs are looking into these complex neurological and systemic conditions.

Some patients with orthopedic conditions and sports injuries who have undergone these treatments have seen promising results. At the same time, there are also patients who have not seen much response. Patient all heal differently, and the extent of their condition can vary. Inconsistent outcomes are due to a lack of standardized stem cell treatment procedures.

A Word About Platelet-Rich Plasma

To add even more complexity, there are other procedures such as the well-known platelet-rich plasma therapy. This is the extraction of platelets from your blood. The platelets contain several different compounds with an anti-inflammatory effect on the local cells. There are 20 different ways of making PRP, of which 17 are bogus! Also, PRP injected in the joint versus in soft tissues, such as muscle or plantar fascia, may behave very differently and may require a different preparation within the same patient.

The biggest misconception about PRP has been that it can by itself be regenerative. Or that PRP alone is stem cell therapy. As noted earlier in the chapter, your blood does not contain any stem cells. PRP is good for reducing inflammation naturally. But if you are dealing with significant tissue loss, you will need actual stem cells to promote regrowth. Too often, athletes are only given a PRP injection and expected to heal and recover completely. This will not happen with the use of PRP alone. Think of stem cells as the seeds and PRP as a good fertilizer. PRP by itself is *not* stem cell therapy.

A2M

A recently identified protein in your blood is called A2M (alpha-2-macroglobulin). This protein can help negate the effect of toxic enzymes that destroy your cartilage. Cartilage lines the surface of the ends of the bones forming the joint. It's like the tread on your car tire. With time and mileage on your joints, the cartilage in the joints starts to wear out. A2M therapy is again not stem cell therapy by itself. The effectiveness of A2M is currently being evaluated.

Exosomes

These are tiny bubbles released by cells that can contain various compounds. Exosomes provide an important channel for inter-cellular communication, by which two cells talk to each other. Again, they are not stem cells by themselves. Their exact role in stem cell treatments has yet to be identified.

No Two Stem Cell Treatments Are the Same

Your condition, extent of damage, and the expected outcome should determine your treatment protocol. There is currently a lack of standardization regarding how many cells would be effective in defining your treatment. With medications, we have reached a sense of dosing. And we have a fairly good idea of which patients can benefit from what dosage of a medication.

With stem cells we have no such guidance yet. A general thought process is the more stem cells injected, the better. However, this may not be necessarily true. Similarly, there is no consensus about how many treatments will be needed. Treatment of tennis elbow with stem cells cannot be compared with stem cell treatment for diabetes or kidney failure.

The bottom line is to start focusing more on regeneration and repair rather than just symptomatic relief. Being able to avoid toxic medications or disabling surgery should be the goal. Each one of the various stem cell treatments is a step in that direction. Each stem cell therapy has its limitations. Foreign sources are manipulated by adding chemicals or preservatives and must be frozen in storage. The consequences of such manipulations are not known to us completely at this time. Your own cells are the safest. They come without any risk of introducing a foreign disease or foreign chemical into your body. However, a frequent caveat is that even your own stem cell treatment protocols are not standardized. Two autologous stem cell treatments cannot be compared in their entirety.

But stem cells have to be isolated from their sources in order to be effective. Injecting the tissue by itself without isolating the stem cells first is *not* stem cell treatment. It has the potential of causing more harm than good.

A good way to think of stem cell procedures is to compare various sources of fruit! Say you decide to consume pomegranate. You can have the whole fruit, cold-pressed juice, or juice from concentrates. Or you can have a pomegranate-flavored drink. Technically, you consumed pomegranate. But all of those are not the same and each will have a different potency, just as there are different stem cells and each type will affect your body differently. Finding the right one will be your most important challenge. Our hope is that now that you have some idea about the range of stem cells available, you are better informed to make those decisions.

Stem Cell Collection, Preparation, and Delivery

No matter the source of stem cells, each has to be collected, processed, and made ready for delivery into your body. This can be extremely challenging, requiring precision. How these processes are handled will impact the results you are likely to see after your treatment. Currently available stem cell collection and preparation methods include the following three procedures:

1. Collected, isolated, and injected the same day. (No laboratory manipulation is involved.) Most common when using your own stem cells.
2. Collected and sent to a laboratory for isolation and/or expansion. Then injected another day. Most common when using foreign stem cells.

3. Collected and sent to a laboratory for isolation. Then programmed to grow into a particular kind of cell (induced pluripotent stem cell, or iPSC).

With proper techniques, any type of stem cells can be frozen and stored for future use. How that impacts their efficacy and viability is yet unknown. For your own stem cells, we believe your own body is the best place to store them. However, stem cell treatments are different for different conditions. The best method that will address your specific condition must be followed.

When it comes to the delivery of stem cells, one fundamental rule is known. The stem cells have to reach the site of damage, injury, or disease to be most effective. How that is accomplished depends on the condition being treated and the treatment protocol being used. IV, or intravenous, cells are not going to reach the inside of your joint, or for that matter your brain. How will the injury heal? Direct injection into the site of injury or damage is still the best bet for getting results with stem cell therapy. For certain conditions, intravenous, intra-arterial, inhalation, intranasal, and intrathecal (CSF) are being studied and evaluated.

As far as your bones and joints are concerned, direct delivery of cells into the area of damage or injury is most effective. A lot of these treatments can be performed through a tiny needle using imaging guidance such as ultrasound or X-ray. It is important to reach the area where stem cell help is needed. The recovery is quick. There are no skin incisions or stitches to deal with.

Stem Cell Pillars of Success

Unlike medications and drugs, stem cells are not an off-the-shelf treatment, although some commercial suppliers are trying to make it so. Stem cells have to be handled with care. A series of steps are involved in preparing stem cells for your treatment. Each step is complex and demands utmost expertise.

When it comes to any stem cell treatments, there are three essential steps that need to be done correctly. These steps are critically important in order for you to get enough stem cells. Unless performed precisely, stem cell treatment won't be effective—a frustration shared by many who do not see results.

The three important pillars of success in stem cell treatments are:

1. Proper harvesting of stem cells sources
2. Correct separation of stem cells from the source
3. Precise delivery of stem cells to the area where help is needed

If any of these three steps is not performed correctly, it can impact the outcome following the procedure. All three steps may be performed in the same-day, same-sitting procedure. This is done generally when your own stem cells are utilized. The steps may be completed on different days, especially when foreign sources of stem cells are being used or if your own cells are being reprogrammed. How each of the three steps will be performed should also be dictated by the condition that is being treated.

A Word of Caution!

Too often, we rush into treatments without establishing a proper diagnosis first. It is important that before any treatment is planned and long before you even consider stem cell treatment as an option, you should have a proper diagnosis and know what you're dealing with. Stem cells offer another powerful tool that can help you heal, provided your condition requires stem cells. Do not choose stem cell treatment just because it's a fad.

A lot of stem cell treatments are new, and scientific evidence may be lacking. In order to consider a stem cell treatment, there must be some scientific basis for how it can help you. You can then decide, based on the science, if and which stem cell treatment is right for you. As noted before, foreign sources may come with the risk of safety, viability, rejection, infection, and disease transmission. Your own cells have the lowest risk associated with them. Once you decide that stem cells are the best solution, you need to make sure there's a good way of delivering them to the area in your body where help is needed. Stem cell viability (how many were alive) is also extremely important and should be documented. This will help in evaluating your results and also planning additional stem cell treatments if needed. Beware of false advertisements. If it sounds too good to be true, it's likely not true. You should have clear answers to fundamental questions before you spend time and money.

KEY TAKEAWAYS

Questions to ask:

1. How will stem cells help your particular condition? Remember, when it comes to stem cell treatments, one size does not fit all!
2. What is the source of the stem cells being given to you? Foreign versus your own stem cells? Risks and benefits?
3. How many stem cells are you getting? The number of live stem cells (not just a total count) you are actually getting is important.
4. How will the stem cells be delivered into your site of injury or damage or area where help is needed? Does the delivery route make sense?
5. If the stem cells were programmed or stored in a laboratory, what preservatives or other agents were added to them? How will that impact their effectiveness and possible long-term side effects?
6. Are you getting PRP (platelet rich plasma)? By itself, this is not "stem cell therapy."

CHAPTER 5

Stem Cells and Joint Pain

What good is a functioning mind and a beating heart

if we cannot move?

Move Your Body

CASE STUDY: **LINDA**

Linda is a pleasant 50-year-old woman, unfortunately afflicted with childhood polio. She has paralysis of her right leg. Linda has been using an assistive device to walk and move since the injury. She has raised two daughters and worked all her life, despite severe physical limitations. Over the past few years, she started to notice pain in her left "good" knee. Linda has gone the usual route of anti-inflammatories. But in spite of meds, the pain has gradually increased. Interestingly, the right knee joint in her affected leg looks structurally intact. Yet she's never been able to put much weight on it. The knee in her polio-affected leg escaped the rigors of daily wear and tear. However, all of the burden has impacted the left knee. It is now showing signs of excessive wear, tear, and degeneration.

Her left knee injury has accelerated faster than what would occur in someone using both knees. Last year Linda was advised that she needed knee joint replacement surgery. She faces the dilemma of a major surgery. If something went wrong during the knee joint replacement surgery, her only good leg could become immobile. There are real risks associated with joint replacement surgery. These risks include bleeding, infection, and blood clots, to name a few. There may also be a need for a revision surgery in a few years. Clearly, a better solution should be offered to Linda to help her save her joint.

Common Causes of Chronic Joint Pain

"We have all experienced joint pain in some shape or form. The most common cause is due to wear and tear of the joint as we age. This is called "degenerative joint disease." It is also popularly labeled "osteoarthritis." Excessive and overuse of our joints without proper rest leads to chronic pain. Conversely, lack of exercise, obesity, and poor diet and nutrition can also lead to painful joints. The underlying reason for pain is inflammation that sets in at the cellular level.

Approximately two out of every three people above the age of 50 may have some degenerative changes affecting one or more joints. As people age, their joints start to become painful without any apparent reason. But, of course, there is a reason, and it has to do with the cartilage covering the ends of the bones, which provides the cushion that helps us stay active. Gradually, as we age, the cartilage starts to become thinner. Repeated stress on the joints causes lining to wear off. The underlying bones are exposed, and the joints start to become more painful with activity. Morning stiffness sets in, and common daily activities become difficult. Common joints affected are hips, knees, shoulders, lower back, fingertips, and even the root of the thumbs. Like several other conditions, the severity of degenerative changes in the joints is also influenced by genetics—your family history.

Another form of joint inflammation is rheumatoid arthritis, although much less common. It is different from degenerative arthritis and may occur much sooner in life. Rheumatoid arthritis causes your own cells to attack cartilage, causing the cartilage to be destroyed. Women are affected by rheumatoid arthritis more than men. The joints become painful and swollen. Joints on both sides of the body are affected. These include wrists, knees, hands, and ankles. Because rheumatoid arthritis involves your own body attacking your own cells, organs such as the heart, lungs, and skin may also be affected. Rheumatoid arthritis is an autoimmune disorder with no definitive cure.

Another cause of painful joints is gout. When crystals of uric acid (a waste by-product from your body normally expelled in the urine) get accumulated in the joint space, they cause inflammation and pain. Gout is more common in obese men who are heavy drinkers. Excessive amounts of seafood and red meat can also increase deposition of uric acid. Poor kidney function and family history can contribute. Just like other forms of arthritis, gout symptoms can wax and wane over a period of time.

Avascular necrosis (AVN) is another condition that can cause joint pain. As the name suggests, lack of adequate blood supply causes inflammation in our bones, ultimately leading to cell death. It can show up without warning. Commonly affected joints are at the hip, wrist, and ankle. The pain can be excruciating. Any movement at the involved joint becomes extremely painful and limited. What causes AVN may not be readily apparent. It can be seen in undiagnosed fractures, exacerbated with excessive alcohol use and the use of steroids. Steroids, whether taken systemically or locally injected and applied, can have devastating side effects. AVN has been reported even with extremely short-term use of steroids. Other causes of AVN include lupus, sickle cell disease, and radiation therapy.

Mainstream Treatments

No matter the cause of joint pain, they all lead to progressive destruction of the joint surfaces and worsening pain. There is no actual cure for most conditions affecting your joints. As symptoms progress, you seek relief. This is mainly in the form of suppressing your symptoms. NSAIDs, cortisone or gel injections, physical therapy, and arthroscopy are generally recommended, one after the other. The concern with these treatments is that they do not address the underlying continued destruction of your joints. At best, they try to control the symptoms. Invariably your pain almost always returns after a brief period. Physical therapy in the presence of an inflamed and severely degenerated joint can be counterproductive and cause you more harm. Your joint continues to deteriorate further. As pain becomes more severe, joint replacement becomes your only option.

Toxic Treatments

Steroids are toxic to our cells. Surprisingly, when a steroid or cortisone injection is given inside a joint, the medication can still be absorbed into the rest of your body. This can cause systemic problems. For example, it can increase your blood sugar levels. For patients with diabetes, sugar control becomes a challenge.

Providing another challenge, arthroscopic surgery generally involves a wash and cleaning of your joint. As simple as it may sound, this process alone can cause significant inflammation. In addition, arthroscopy may involve removing some meniscus and cartilage (the cushions in the joint), thereby leaving your joint in a weaker state. Furthermore, studies have shown that immobilization following surgery can itself be detrimental to your joints.

Clearly, we need better treatments. Mainstream medicine has only offered temporary relief. Often your joint continues to degenerate until it becomes so painful and nonfunctional, you are left with no choice. Joint pain takes its toll in the impact it has on the quality of your life and in lost time. Studies have even linked depression to knee pain. Months and years go by as your activities continue to decline. This is the biggest price you pay with joint pain—not being able to do the things and activities you enjoy.

CASE STUDY: **MS. HERNANDEZ**

Ms. Hernandez, a Jehovah's Witness, is a 67-year-old grandmother who lives with pain. The pain in her hip joints has become increasingly worse over the past few months. She received a cortisone injection in her hip joints a few months ago. She had some pain relief for a week. But then the pain came back with a vengeance. She has been told she needs hip replacement surgery. Hip replacement surgery is associated with significant blood loss. This is a problem because Jehovah's Witnesses do not accept blood transfusions, nor do they believe in donating or storing their own blood for transfusion purposes. There are some products, one being stem cells, that Jehovah's Witnesses can accept as long as no other blood cells are present.

There are many others like Ms. Hernandez, suffering in private. Besides religious beliefs, the fear and the consequences of surgery leave them with no options. Loss of mobility leads to depression. Joint pain has ramifications beyond just the injured. It takes a toll on family members and caregivers.

Role of Stem Cells

Stem cells can promote replication and regeneration due to their three important properties. They are anti-inflammatory. They can modify the environment of the local cells by removing toxic chemicals and unhealthy cells. And stem cells improve the circulation to local cells by forming new blood vessels. Currently available stem cells rely on these properties to help promote regeneration and repair. In addition, stem cells secrete valuable growth factors that promote regeneration and repair. They hold great promise, although further research is needed.

The lack of standardization is also a big hurdle. Stem cell treatment by itself is just a "title." It doesn't tell you what kind of treatment you are likely to receive. The devil is in the details! It is important to understand broad differences among various types and sources of stem cells. This can help you make an informed decision when it comes to choosing a treatment.

Available Methods of Stem Cell Therapy That May Alleviate Joint Pain

Stem Cells Derived from Your Own Body

This generally involves collecting source tissue from your body and then breaking it down to filter your own stem cells. These cells can then be injected into the joint in the same-day, same-sitting procedure. Or they might be sent to a laboratory for further cleaning along with expansion or multiplication.

Commonly utilized source tissues are bone marrow and fat. It is very important to make a fundamental clarification here. Every organ system of your body can be a source of stem cells. Fat and bone marrow are easily dispensable sources that surgeons have been harvesting for many years. The techniques for harvesting these tissues are fairly refined. Removal of fat and bone marrow, even in significant amounts, does not negatively impact your body. Therefore, these two sources by default have become the most common sources for getting your own stem cells.

There is another way your own tissue can be utilized. A portion of cartilage from your joint can be removed and then grown in a laboratory. This can create more cartilage, which can then be surgically implanted back into the joint. Of course, unlike a simple injection with stem cells, cartilage implants require extensive surgery.

CASE STUDY: **MICHAEL AND JOYCE**

Michael and his wife, Joyce, are both in their mid-60s. They love to go heli-skiing every year. Both suffer from chronic knee pain. Both have been recommended knee surgery multiple times. They have also been told to stop heli-skiing. Thrashing their knees for 20 days in the mountains isn't good for knee recovery. Still, they won't do it. They love skiing and won't give it up. They have taken care of their bodies. Outside of their heli-ski passion, nearly every moment is devoted to their grandkids. Every two years Michael and Joyce get an injection of their own stem cells into their knees. This maintains good tissue and repairs worn-out tissue. Stem cell therapy keeps them active as they continue to enjoy their passion. They maximize the very precious time left to spend with their grandkids.

Foreign Sources of Stem Cells

As mentioned in other chapters, stem cells can come from another adult human being, a newborn baby, or a pregnant mother's womb. Since the cells are foreign to your body, there is a risk of rejection. There is also the risk of disease transmission depending on how thoroughly the donor has been screened. Common cells under this category are amniotic, placental, or umbilical cord cells, sometimes collectively called "baby cells." These cells are kept frozen until ready for use.

It is not clear if the process of freezing and thawing prior to injection causes some cells to die. Some cells may also be expanded or replicated in the laboratory. How that impacts the effectiveness of these stem cells is yet unknown. It is important to remember that pure embryonic stem cells, capable of growing into anything, are banned outside of well-regulated clinical trials at academic centers. Let no one fool you on that.

Dangers of Stem Cells

CASE STUDY: **KAREN**

Karen is a 50-year-old real estate agent suffering from low back pain. She totally believes in holistic care and in taking care of her body. She had suffered a back injury years ago, and it is now taking a toll on her daily life. A couple of disks in her lower back have degenerated and were found to be contributing to her pain. She has refused surgery. Karen has been reading a lot about stem cell treatments and is excited about the possibility. She visited two clinics advertising stem cells for the back. At one of the clinics, the doctor was an anesthesiologist who mentioned that umbilical cord cells would be helpful. Karen was also told that her own cells are too weak and are unlikely to produce any benefit. The umbilical cord cells were cleaned and tested for infectious disease. Karen underwent the treatment and felt good for about a week. She then came down with a fever, and her back pain increased. One night she had intense fever and chills followed by nausea and vomiting. Karen had to be rushed to the ER and hospitalized. Following her blood tests, she underwent a CAT scan and an MRI. All the blood tests came back positive for infection in her blood, and as well, the scans showed a large abscess in the area of the stem cell injection.

This is again a reminder that we're not at the stage where stem cell safety is 100%. Especially when a foreign source is involved, there can be major risks. The questions to ask are:

- Where were the cord cells collected?
- Which women were the donors?
- Did these women consent to donating their baby's cord for stem cells?
- How thorough was the history and laboratory testing to rule out infectious agents in the donated cord tissue?
- How were the stem cells cleaned and processed?
- How will the stem cells be delivered for injection into your body?

There are no definitive answers to any of these questions. All these steps involved in stem cell treatments are not well regulated. At this time, there is very little oversight of foreign stem cells. You have to be careful.

No medical procedure comes without any risk. It would be naive to believe that stem cells are going to be completely safe. We are at the beginning stages of stem cell treatments. We know very little about them. That is why there has to be an extremely prudent approach in offering stem cell treatments. We do know that the patient's own stem cells might escape rejection. However, there's always the risk of infection and the possibility of tumor formation. If there is a mutation of the DNA or some damage or alteration to the cells, they can have uncontrolled growth, in other words, cancer. Therefore, it's extremely important to understand stem cell therapies. The risk of embryonic stem cells or cells that were manufactured in a laboratory causing infection and tumor formation is even higher. The effect of the various chemicals used in the laboratory during the isolation, cleaning, and programming of stem cells can have far-reaching consequences.

There are stories of patients going blind following stem cell therapy or a nose growing on the patient's back. Some of these stories may be based on facts, and some are just crazy rumors. However, it's extremely important to understand the entire process. You need to understand the nature of the cell source and any laboratory processing that might be involved. You also need to know how the cells will be delivered. It is important to know whether a test can be done on stem cells to reduce the possibility of contamination. Also, you should learn whether the cells have been altered in a manner that may harm you.

The stem cell delivery procedure is much less invasive when compared with surgery. Some stem cells are used in conjunction with surgery. There are some that need to be implanted into the body, requiring an invasive procedure. Most stem cell treatments for joint regeneration and repair are done through a simple injection. The downtime is minimal. Most patients return to active life soon.

A Word About Platelet-Rich Plasma

PRP is derived from you own blood. Your blood has three types of cells: red blood cells that carry oxygen, white blood cells that fight infection, and platelets. Plasma is the fluid of the blood in which these cells are suspended. Once the red blood cells and the white blood cells have been removed from your sample of blood, you are left with PRP. Platelets perform a variety of functions in the body. Most importantly, platelets carry 10 anti-inflammatory and growth factors. PRP has been shown to be superior to both cortisone and hyaluronic acid gel injections in controlling joint pain. Of course, like any other treatment, PRP has its downside. The problem with PRP is twofold:

1. There are 20 different ways of making PRP, 17 of which don't work and won't give you good-quality PRP. Hence the effectiveness of PRP cannot be compared.

2. As we have stated before, PRP by itself is not regenerative. This means if there is actual joint damage, loss of cartilage, or a tear, you need stem cells to grow and repair. PRP is not stem cell therapy. What PRP can do is make stem cell therapy more effective. Also, PRP works great by itself when treating inflammation. Certainly, it is much better than a cortisone injection. Purely inflammatory conditions like plantar fasciitis and tennis elbow can respond well to PRP-only treatments.

A2M Exosomes and Cytokines

A2M exosomes and cytokines are products that can be derived from your body and may have some anti-inflammatory benefits. These newer elements require further study before their routine application can be recommended for joint pain.

Heal Your Body to Heal Your Joint

No matter the treatment, ultimately it's your body that heals you. Starting with a positive mind, maintaining good hydration, and watching sugar intake are critical to a pain-free life. Normal body weight for your height limits the stress your joints are exposed to. Heat therapy is another good tool to help soothe not only your joints but also the ligaments, tendons, and muscles that support them. Ice is good when you have an acute injury; other than that, heat is the way to go. Your daily good habits will serve you better in the long run than any treatment. Even the magic of stem cells will disappear if you are not healthy. Later in the book, we will discuss more in depth about daily habits and rituals you can follow to be healthier and more pain-free.

CASE STUDY: **MR. COOPER**

Mr. Cooper is a 65-year-old professional piano player and teacher. Over the years, joints in his right thumb have become painful. Having taken anti-inflammatories for years, he now uses a brace on his thumb to minimize the pain. However, the pain is becoming more and more unbearable. Mr. Cooper has a large following of students and really loves teaching. He was advised that he will need hand fusion surgery. His thumb joints would be fused together with a metal plate and screws. This would effectively end his performances and speed his retirement from the piano.

That is a worst-case scenario. He is still in extremely good health and wants to continue with his passion. Dejected, Mr. Cooper shared the dilemma with his students. He was disappointed at the prospect of not teaching and developing these rising stars. One of the students' mothers, an avid tennis player, told him that she had had stem cell treatments for both knee joints. After recovery, she was back playing singles four times a week. So Mr. Cooper went to see her doctor. After seeing the doc, Mr. Cooper received the same diagnosis of advanced wear and tear on his thumb joints. He was told that a series of treatments using his own stem cells will be needed in order to regenerate and repair the damage. He also was told that the pain, after a few months of rehab, could be reduced to a level where he should be able to play the piano fairly comfortably. Mr. Cooper understands that stem cell treatments would not make his joints normal again. However, with some relief, he could continue his passion. Continuing what he loved would be a dream come true.

These treatments are by no means a recommendation. A lot more data need to be collected, much more research needs to be done, and standardization needs to be achieved. The FDA has not yet approved the treatments. Interestingly, regulatory bodies of every country view them differently. Some countries have taken the lead and may have already approved them. Check with your doctor about the most recent regulatory status and any concerns.

Our goal is to give you an idea of the various therapies available. You should do your due diligence in evaluating them. Ask questions and understand what kind of stem cell therapy you are getting. The cost and number of treatment sessions may vary. Also check with your local regulatory authorities about the status of these treatments in your area. There are so many variations in stem cell treatments. Some not approved in one country may be approved in another. The essential takeaway here is that while stem cells will play an important role in preserving your joints, much work needs to be done to further understand both the potential of stem cells and their limitations.

KEY TAKEAWAYS

1. Merely masking the symptoms won't control damage to your joints.
2. Maintain normal body weight.
3. Cut down sugar intake.
4. Heat therapy is best for chronic pain.
5. Understand the role of stem cells in treating joint pain.

CHAPTER 6

Stem Cells and Back Pain

You don't have to live with back pain.

End the Suffering

Back pain affects all age groups. It is a worldwide leading cause of lost productivity. A wide range of treatments is usually prescribed. These consist of rest, anti-inflammatories, injections, and surgery. Often the outcomes are poor. None focus on addressing the root causes. They only attempt to calm the symptoms. It is always important to understand what causes back pain in the first place.

CASE STUDY: TOM

Tom is a 48-year-old businessman who lived almost half of his life with back pain. Tom was very active in his college days playing football and basketball and was heavily (no pun intended) into weightlifting. Tom was as healthy and fit as they come, having the time of his life. Then the unexpected happened. At 24, he first experienced back pain. Tom noticed an intense pain starting in his lower back and shooting down the back of his leg. He sought the advice of his primary care doctor. Tom was told he most likely had sciatica and was advised to rest. Pain medications such as Ibuprofen and Naprosyn were also prescribed.

Tom found some relief from these medications but could not completely shake off the pain. A month passed, and he was still feeling miserable. During his follow-up appointment, Tom expressed concern that the pain was continuing. He was frustrated with the inability to engage in his favorite activities. His physician prescribed stronger pain meds and said the pain would gradually subside. Tom was losing patience. His entire life had been disrupted by back pain. Tom was having a hard time keeping up his daily routine. At work, he was forced to take frequent breaks to get through the day.

He called the physician, stating the pain was worse. Pain medications offered just a few hours of relief. The physician recommended Tom see a physical therapist. That resulted in some exercises, which Tom did diligently. The physical therapy did provide some relief, but the pain returned. About eight weeks into his PT, Tom wasn't improving. He called his doctor, requesting more meds. Tom was refused and was perceived as a drug seeker. Tom's doctor asserted that the back pain should have resolved by now.

Tom's life was turning upside down. He tried making modifications in his work schedule, and even tried switching jobs, but nothing brought him relief. He was becoming a social recluse. He had to find another physician. The new doc ordered an MRI of Tom's lumbar (low back) spine area. The MRI showed disk herniation. The new physician prescribed cortisone injections. Tom received the first injection two days later at an interventional radiologist's office (an interventional radiologist is a physician who specializes in performing minimally invasive procedures under imaging guidance). Tom felt better after the injection. For the next week, he was able to do more activities than when the pain first started.

But by the beginning of the following week, the pain returned with a vengeance. At this point, Tom was in excruciating pain. This time his doc said Tom would need additional cortisone injections. Over the next two months, Tom received four, all providing temporary relief. But the pain always came back.

Desperate to prove he was not a drug seeker, Tom tried to find relief without pain meds. He was eventually referred to a spine surgeon. After a five-minute appointment, Tom got a date for surgery. He was assured by the surgeon that the success rate was very high. Tom looked forward to the relief and desperately wanted to get his life back. However, a month after surgery, the pain returned. The sharpness had decreased, but now he had a new constant dull aching pain in his lower back. He was advised to go for physical therapy again with a promise that the pain would diminish.

Over the past 24 years, Tom had four spinal surgeries. Yet the outcome hasn't been good. He still lives with back pain.

Unfortunately, Tom's case is not very different from that of scores of others. What can you do if you suffer from back pain? Certainly, your posture is central. No wonder postural adjustments and exercises have shown to be one of the most effective interventions in managing back pain. Next, your general health, body weight, and body mass index play an important part, and finally the medications you take. Be wary of meds. Drugs can contribute to your back pain and in some cases make it worse.

Causes of Back Pain

There are a number of causes of back pain. Unfortunately, the most common causes are often missed or their role underestimated.

Spinal Disks

One cause is the degeneration of the spinal disks. The intervertebral disks are like cushions between the bony block vertebral bodies that stack on top of each other forming your spinal column. This "cushion" thins out, stressing the vertebral bodies. This causes back pain. These cushions are also important because they help maintain a healthy space between the bony vertebral bodies. Maintaining that space is extremely important. This is where the nerves come out from the spinal cord. If the cushion between the bony elements becomes thinner, there is more pressure on the nerves due to the tightening of the space available. This causes pain to often cascade down arms or legs.

Another mechanism making life miserable is developing tears, bulges, or disk herniation. This simply means that disk material extends out of its confined space. While some herniation can occur by lifting something heavy, most herniations develop in disks that have worn out and are degenerated. Depending on the location, the herniated disk can press on the surrounding nerves, causing either worsening central back pain or sciatica that cascades down arms and legs. By this time, your spine has taken a lot of beating. Your ability to lead a productive life has diminished.

Facet Joint Back Pain

Another underestimated cause is degenerative changes in the facet joints. Facet joints are the small joints that connect the bony vertebral bodies as they stack one on top of another. Facet joints facilitate motions in our back. They help us lean, bend, turn, and twist. If there were no facet joints, your back would be one rigid column! So just like the knee or shoulder or any other joint, facet joints wear out. Because the joints are located toward the back portion of the bony vertebral bodies, pain is often more pronounced when you arch the spine backward. As wear and tear progresses, the facet joints can become arthritic, again just like any other joint.

Myofascial and Ligament Pain

The muscles and ligaments surrounding the spine are designed to support posture and other complex movements. They make movement effortless so that we can enjoy activities. It is extremely important these muscles and ligaments are kept healthy through regular exercise. Stretching and resistance training are important to keep your paraspinal muscles and ligaments strong to support your spine.

Vertebral Body Fracture and Compression Fracture

Vertebral compression fractures are rarely traumatic. They are generally more likely as we age. The bones become weaker. Even daily routine activities can cause compression fractures. The worst part is that they can be extremely painful. The whole stack of vertebral bodies can cause significant pressure on the fractured level, making even minimal motions extremely painful. Surprisingly, this condition is becoming more common in younger populations—especially in patients who have been subjected to cortisone and steroid therapy. Steroids are powerful chemicals that, as mentioned above, can make your bones weaker.

Compression fractures have no real treatment. Most patients end up in the emergency room because of the pain and are put on pain medications. Pain and discomfort in the first few weeks can be very debilitating. Besides compression fracture discomfort, pain med side effects make life miserable. Fractures eventually heal. But as they do, bones deform, putting other vertebral bodies at risk. Surgically stabilizing the spine would be too invasive and a horrible choice.

CASE STUDY: **TRACY**

Tracy is a 40-year-old woman who has dealt with asthma most of her life. One day she felt pain in her lower back. She consulted a pain management physician and was prescribed strong medications. After a few weeks without any significant relief, she was given epidural injections. Another few weeks went by, and yet Tracy's pain persisted. At this point, she consulted another physician, who ordered an MRI of her spine. The MRI showed the presence of a compression fracture within a vertebral body. When one of these bony squares fractures and becomes deformed, the whole column becomes unstable.

Vertebral body compression fractures are usually seen in elderly postmenopausal women. They happen in response to the loss of bone structure. This bone thinning is called "osteopenia." In advanced stages, it progresses into osteoporosis. Because bone is weak, very little pressure or trauma can cause these fractures. Normal routine daily activities can contribute to fractures.

However, Tracy's case was different. She was still young and didn't fit the profile of someone who would suffer from this condition. Unfortunately, Tracy was already receiving corticosteroid treatments in an attempt to manage her asthma. Steroids can lead to loss of bone structure and premature bone weakness.

Besides steroids, certain antacids and antibiotics can also cause weak bones.

A treatment called "kyphoplasty" can help. Few patients know about this procedure. It involves placing a small needle in the compressed vertebra. A balloon is inserted through the needle, elevating the compression fracture deformity. This is followed by the placement of bone cement into the vertebral body to help maintain its shape. Pain relief can be immediate. But none of this addresses the root problem, which is thinning of the bone.

Following a diet rich in calcium, exercising regularly, keeping well hydrated, and avoiding medications that lead to bone loss are all important strategies to consider. This is another area where it is hoped that stem cells will have a role to play in the near future. Stem cells can help fractures heal and also make bones stronger. There is still a lot to learn about the use of stem cells to treat back problems. More studies are needed to document their safety and the specific role stem cells can play.

CASE STUDY: **ERICA**

Erica was an 18-year-old high school gymnast when she started experiencing tightness and stiffness in her lower back. The greatest discomfort was after workouts. At first, she ignored it. She hoped rest might make the pain go away. She started taking over-the-counter anti-inflammatories. Soon she had trouble getting out of bed in the morning. She was advised to undergo physical therapy and take some time out from gymnastics. Erica completed a two-month course of physical therapy and avoided the sport she loved so much. Even so, pain increased in her lower back. The physician told Erica and her parents that she was having some psychological issues. The pain was all in her head. Obviously, this made Erica's parents even more concerned. They suspected the problem was a reaction to stress. This frustrated Erica because she was dealing with real pain. It now seemed like nobody believed her. She was even forced to see a psychotherapist before her doctor would give her any more pain meds. Erica's pain continued. She could barely keep up with her daily routine.

The pain medications also caused nausea, so much so, that Erica hated taking them. Her doctor prescribed steroids to reduce the inflammation. As a result of the steroids and a lack of physical exercise, Erica gained 20 pounds in three months. If she didn't have depression before, she did now. She was also referred to a chiropractor specializing in spinal manipulation. He tried to align her back, but the manipulation instead significantly increased her pain. When she returned to the chiropractor the following day, she was told to be patient. The pain would go away. Erica was advised to continue more sessions of spinal manipulation.

Over the next few months, she saw multiple physical therapists. She also had acupuncture therapies. Nothing gave her relief. She was becoming disabled. Her health insurance finally allowed a spine surgeon visit. The specialist immediately ordered X-rays, a CT scan, and an MRI of the lumbar spine. The results showed a tiny fracture in her lower spine leading to forward slippage of her vertebral body. The condition is known as spondylolysis with spondylolisthesis. Finally, after 18 months, Erica had a diagnosis. Now a treatment could be planned. She had been suffering from a real spine problem. The pain was not in her head. Unfortunately, she did not need to suffer for all these months. Her young life was wrecked.

Sacroiliac Joint Involvement

Sacroiliac (SI) joint involvement is another often missed cause of low back pain. As many as one in four cases of low back pain could be due to SI joint dysfunction. It can feel similar to sciatica. In SI the sacroiliac joints connect the pelvis to the lower portion of the spine, called the "sacrum." These joints help absorb shock and the weight from the upper body down to the legs. SI joint dysfunction can be caused by either too little or too much movement. Often seen in young adults and women following pregnancy, stiffness and pain are two important symptoms. In advanced stages, instability of gait can develop.

Drugs Can Cause Back Pain

A frequent cause of back pain may be lurking in your medicine cabinet. Your pain could be a result of the medications you take. You can experience back pain from certain antibiotics, cholesterol-lowering drugs, blood pressure and diabetes pills, and asthma medications. Even certain drugs used to treat osteoporosis—drugs you take for strengthening your bones—can cause back pain! One should always be aware that commonly prescribed medications can often be the culprits.

Referred Causes of Back Pain

Referred pain is pain felt in one area due to a problem in another area. In other words, the underlying cause is not where you feel the pain, but instead the cause is located in another part of your body. For example, kidney stones, infection, AAA (abdominal aortic aneurysm), gallstones, and uterine fibroids and other pelvic conditions in women can all cause back pain.

Tumors and cancers can develop in the spine and cause low back pain. So can infection in the spine, especially if your immune system is weak.

Congenital or birth-related defects can also cause back pain. Common among these is abnormal curvature of the spine. This causes the spine to abnormally bend in one or more particular directions. Scoliosis is when the spine bends excessively sideways. A backward bend creating a hump is called "kyphosis." A forward bend is called "lordosis." Each one of these makes the spine unstable and can lead to back pain, especially in the young and otherwise healthy.

Spina bifida is a birth defect that occurs when bones of the spine are not fully fused. A tethered cord means that a spinal cord is attached usually to the base of the spine, or tailbone, by an inelastic tissue. This creates pain every time you try to bend forward or hold some weight at the level of the waist. While most cases are due to birth-related defects, a tethered cord can also develop in adults, especially if you have undergone previous spine surgery.

When to Treat and When Not To

CASE STUDY: **ROGER**

Roger, a 62-year-old golfer, suffered from knee arthritis for several years. He had been managing it with painkillers, cortisone injections, and hyaluronic acid as well as gel injections. Over the last few months, Roger noticed increasing low back pain. His surgeons recommended knee joint replacement surgery. Roger wanted to delay it as long as possible. Perhaps even avoid surgery altogether. However, the low back pain was causing a lot of concern. Roger was not willing to accept his body breaking down.

He sought the advice of a doctor specializing in regenerative treatments of joints and spine. After a detailed clinical exam in which Roger had to lie down, stand up, and walk, it was determined that his back pain was caused by his knees. Roger had been living with this painful condition for a long time. No mainstream treatments were making the situation any better. In an attempt to avoid knee pain, Roger's body compensated with a pelvic tilt (lopsided pelvis). This put a strain on his lower back.

Roger underwent regenerative stem cell therapy on both knees. Within three months, his knee pain decreased and his activity level had improved. And he no longer had back pain.

This is the advantage that stem cells can offer. They can regenerate and repair. They can help cut off the chain reaction of pain that develops when a problem in one area affects another area.

This also suggests a need to seek help early. Until now, patients with back and joint pain have resisted seeking help. Mainstream treatment options are dismal. Nobody looks forward to toxic medications. Nobody wants to consider the body-destroying steroids and the risk of disabling surgeries. But now you have an option. You now can consider regenerative stem cell therapy that truly can help preserve your body.

Back Pain and Regeneration

Provided the correct diagnosis is made early on, there are several causes of back pain that can be managed effectively. A spectrum of stem cell treatments has been shown to be effective in regenerating the disk and repairing facet joints. These treatments can make healthy mobility possible without pain. Look into these treatments before considering physical therapy or surgery. Help early on can prevent years of misery.

Stem cell therapy is not a cure for everything in the spine. If you have certain problems involving nerves, current stem cell treatment may not have a role in ameliorating the pain. The problem could be a severely herniated disk that is pressing on the nerve roots, or it might be a tumor making your spine unstable. Stem cells are not at the point where they have any role in helping with these conditions. So do not waste your time and money risking your health. If you have these conditions, you will most likely need surgery.

If you are an otherwise healthy middle-aged adult, get help as soon as you feel back pain. Don't ignore the early symptoms. Most of these are due to disk degeneration or facet joint arthritis or a combination of both. The cushions of the disk are the places where stem cells can help in repair and regeneration. Stem cells can rebuild the surfaces of the facet joints, allowing your spine to maintain flexibility. The stem cell treatment for back pain is new but promising. More research is needed to document its safety and long-term efficacy. Get treatment before you start having neurological symptoms like nerve compression or pinching and shooting pain. When you experience these symptoms, the damage has progressed so far that there may be few options left.

Spine surgery is not the answer. With surgery comes scar tissue formation. Scar tissue can replace your original pain with new pain! Take care of your body. Your posture and daily exercise are equally important to maintaining a healthy spine. Hydration is essential. Learn to manage your back with daily routines like stretching, massage, heat therapy, sauna, and steam. Your exercises should focus in particular on building the paraspinal muscles. The job of the paraspinal muscles is to support your spine as it bends, twists, and turns. The paraspinal muscles allow you to move in one direction and recover to another. If your spine is not properly supported by the surrounding muscles, you will continue to suffer back pain.

KEY TAKEAWAYS

1. Seek proper diagnosis early! Don't let rest, medications, or physical therapy mask the problem. You must know what the underlying cause is before you start on a treatment plan.
2. Remember, your problem may not be in your back. Seek various opinions.
3. A proper exercise routine focused on strengthening paraspinal muscles is key to lifelong spinal health. Exercise before you develop a problem!
4. Stay hydrated every day. This is the cheapest investment you can make in keeping back pain at bay.
5. Stem cells and PRP are rapidly developing tools that can help manage your back pain. Seek more information.

CHAPTER 7

Stem Cells
and Sports Injuries

Turn your setbacks into comebacks!

Don't Just Play. Perform

Sports injury is an important area of success in stem cell therapy.

CASE STUDY: **JESSICA**

Jessica at 12 years old was a competitive swimmer. She injured her knee while colliding with another swimmer in a supposedly noncontact sport. She underwent arthroscopic surgery at a local children's hospital. Unfortunately, she continued to experience pain a year after surgery. After going through rehab, she was unable to do any physical activities, let alone competitive swimming. Her repeated questions to the surgeon went unanswered. She was told everything had gone well with the surgery.

Desperate to find a solution, her parents consulted multiple orthopedic and sports medicine doctors. They all told the parents that Jessica would require corticosteroid injections and possibly another surgery. The worst news for Jessica was that she may not be able to swim competitively ever again. Imagine your child, or any other family member, being told of that outcome, especially if your child is full of promise and is talented and is hoping to make sports a part of his or her life.

Teenage years are such a formative time that any significant event can leave a mark for a lifetime. Soon, Jessica's parents noticed she was unable to sleep at night. She became tired and lethargic during the day. Her academic performance started to suffer. After a year, Jessica was unable even to walk without pain. Her parents happened upon a physician in the community who specialized in stem cell treatments, training, and research.

They scheduled a consultation. After an extensive clinical examination of Jessica's knee, this physician asked her to walk and attempt to run in his office. He wanted to fully understand the extent of her problem. Jessica was impressed by the thorough examination, which also included an ultrasound performed by the physician himself. The doctor then discussed the entire spectrum of stem cell treatments. The family learned about blood cells, platelet-rich plasma (PRP), platelet-poor plasma (PPP), bone marrow cells, fat-derived stem cells (MSC), embryonic cells, umbilical cord cells, and placental and amniotic cells. They discussed the differences between Jessica's own natural cells and foreign-sourced cells.

Even though initial impressions tell us stem cell therapy can be safe, we know very little about how they may behave. Jessica's parents were skeptical about the efficacy. These treatments are so new. They aren't even covered by insurance or approved by the FDA. But the science behind stem cells made so much sense. The family walked away with a wealth of knowledge. For the first time in a year, they had hope that their daughter might recover. Jessica didn't really have any other options. The thought of her using steroids or undergoing another surgery just didn't seem right. What she had done so far would only cause more damage to her knee.

Jessica and her parents decided to use her own blood cells. Two weeks later Jessica underwent a procedure in the physician's office. The cells were delivered precisely with the guidance of both X-rays and ultrasound. After the therapy, the physician prescribed a regimen of non-weight-bearing activities for two weeks. Walking on a level surface was encouraged. In the first two weeks following the procedure, Jessica's pain started to subside. She continued doing the prescribed stretching and lightweight activities over the next two months. At six months Jessica was participating in competitive swimming and track events.

Mainstream Medicine

Mainstream treatments have essentially remained unchanged for the past two decades. The management of sports injuries has largely been confined to a handful of options. It doesn't really matter what part of the body is injured; treatments do not change. Mainstream medicine treats sports injuries with painkillers, steroid injections, and chemicals that cause damage even as they provide temporary relief. They certainly don't help performance. When your injury does not heal, some form of surgery is prescribed leading to a long rehab. A significant loss of playing time is involved.

There is a huge downside to these treatments. That is why there has been such a big push to look at alternatives. How sports injuries are managed can alter the course of an athlete's life. It's extremely important for athletes to get the right kind of care so that they can continue to play their chosen sport for a long time. Athletes and their families sacrifice so much. It's extremely important for them to find the right alternative therapies that can regenerate and repair natural tissue.

Athletes and Sports Injury Diagnosis

CASE STUDY: JOSE

Jose, 56, is an avid soccer player who a year ago was facing surgery because of painful knees. Rather than agreeing to the surgery immediately, he went for a second opinion. Upon a detailed clinical examination, extensive arthritis was found in his hip joint. This caused referred pain to the knee. If Jose's knees had been operated on, the outcome would have been disastrous.

Everybody wants to win, and nobody wants to wait. It is extremely important for athletes to take charge of their own situation.

CASE STUDY: BRANDON

Brandon is a 17-year-old high school football player trying to develop into a great quarterback. He practiced hard looking forward to admission into a top-college football program. When Brandon was 15, he suffered a fall on his right elbow during practice. His right arm was his throwing arm. Brandon complained of some pain, and the team physician advised him to wear a sling for a few weeks.

Brandon was young and thought he could handle the pain. After four weeks, Brandon resumed practice and started to compete again. He was really good, and the team needed him. The team doctors determined that his elbow had healed because the X-rays were negative. During the off-season, Brandon realized that his elbow range of motion was limited. In fact, there were certain movements his elbow couldn't do. Brandon sought an opinion from a physician specializing in regenerative sports medicine. Brandon was told the injury to his elbow was originally a dislocation. Routine X-rays at that age can miss dislocations because the bones are not yet fused. Because Brandon was misdiagnosed, and the proper treatment was not performed, his bones had started to heal abnormally. This led to a deformity limiting his range of motion at his elbow. It especially impacted his throwing ability. Brandon will now need extensive corrective surgery. In the meantime, he has learned to compensate for his deformity.

Younger athletes often don't get the best medical diagnosis. A lot of sports injuries are missed because of conflicting interests between the team winning and the well-being of the athlete. Younger athletes are obviously anxious to prove themselves and please their parents and coaches. They are totally focused on going as far as they can in their chosen sport.

CASE STUDY: **MELISSA**

At 18, Melissa loved playing competitive tennis at a high level. That is, until she developed hip pain. She was a rising tennis star at a renowned academy she had attended since she was

13. Her hip pain was severe, and no relief was in sight. Nothing worked in spite of numerous physical therapy sessions. After a physician at the academy had given her cortisone injections, her pain decreased, but only for a week. When Melissa complained of pain again, her complaint fell on deaf ears. Her coach told her to become mentally tough and learn to deal with it. She was prescribed another three rounds of injections. After that, Melissa never played competitive tennis again.

Today, Melissa still lives with the discomfort of hip pain. During her last orthopedic visit, she was told to start preparing for hip replacement surgery in the next few years. Melissa was only in her late twenties. She dreamed of marrying her longtime boyfriend and one day having a family. But Melissa was worried that she may never be able to again lead a normal life.

Athletes need strong advocates. A pro athlete has an agent. But younger athletes usually suffer without strong protection. But when athletes get injured and become unproductive, they are relegated to the bench. Parents should be the most important advocates for their children. They should seek opinions from physicians outside the team. The goal should be to protect the young athlete.

Sports Injuries and Surgery

Admittedly, some sports injuries do require surgery. At the same time, surgery can be unforgiving. It takes a toll on the body. To repeat the maxim from Chapter 2, the fundamental principle in medicine is, "First, do no harm." Athletes should avoid unnecessary surgery, oral pain meds, and cortisone injections. Surgery can be a severe setback. When you suffer an injury followed by surgery, more problems can be created.

There are clear indications when surgery may be needed. A joint may need to be stabilized. A torn muscle may need to be repaired. A fracture may have to be internally stabilized. But in most cases, surgery adds insult to injury. Twenty years of data have shown that arthroscopic knee surgery can lead to chronic pain and early-onset arthritis.

There are multiple reasons why surgery may not be the answer, especially in chronic conditions. First, surgery is invasive. It can cause collateral damage even when it goes well. Most importantly, surgery is targeted in its approach. It is supposed to fix the main injury. But there could be other associated damage that needs help too.

Imaging studies can only show us so much. There are diagnostic limitations. There is no way of knowing what happens at a cellular level. For example, a patient might have a meniscus tear in the knee causing pain. But what about the loss of cartilage? What about a ligament tear? Surgery will try to fix the meniscus with artificial stitches, although in most knee surgeries, a significant portion of the meniscus ends up getting removed. But other areas contributing to knee pain may not be addressed. Further, the joint will become weaker if tissues such as meniscus or cartilage are removed. Coupled with chronic inflammation at a cellular level, surgery may diminish any meaningful repair and regeneration from occurring.

Ultimately, the development of scar tissue will interfere with performance. "First, do no harm"? Current mainstream medicine has the potential to do more harm than good.

CASE STUDY: **MARK**

Mark is a 40-year-old surfer dealing with pain in the back of his thighs. About three years ago Mark was trying to move furniture around in his house. A large cabinet came loose, and as Mark tried to keep it from falling, his legs slipped from underneath him and he heard a popping sensation behind both his hips. Mark was in severe pain and noticed extensive bruising on the backs of his thighs. He knew something major had gone wrong. He called up his doctor, who asked him to come over to the clinic the next morning. His doctor ordered an MRI examination. The MRI showed that Mark had suffered bilateral hamstring tears. He was referred to an orthopedic surgeon, who advised surgery. The immediate recovery after surgery was uneventful. He started rehab after about a month. Five months out of surgery, Mark had partial pain relief. Still, on some nights, the pain was severe enough to keep him awake.

Besides surfing, Mark loved hitting the wilderness, hiking, and photography. He would feel a sense of peace and calmness going into the wilderness. However, he could do none of that with his pain. Another year had passed by, and yet Mark still couldn't do many outdoor activities. He was starting to feel depressed. He sought the opinion of many other doctors and physical therapists. All said he may need another surgery. Mark was reluctant to go under the knife again. He had been doing regular stretching, massage, sauna, and heat therapy, and that way he could keep his pain under control. But the development of significant scar tissue would limit the extent of his motion.

Mark wanted to get back to doing the activities he loved. Seeing his frustration, one day his chiropractor referred him to a doctor specializing in regenerative sports medicine. Regenerative medicine focuses on regenerating and repairing natural tissues.

Mark was treated with a combination of his own stem cells injected directly into the area of the tears. The scar tissue that had built up following surgery was also targeted. A special technique was used to break down the scar tissue within his muscle. The entire procedure was performed under ultrasound guidance at the physician's office. Mark has had two sessions of treatment and has been pain-free over the past two years. He is back surfing and recently put up a website posting a collection of his photographs taken in the wild.

For many years, elite athletes have traveled to Europe and South America seeking advanced treatments. Stem cells are often associated with celebrities. Some stories are true, while others are fake. But the real question is why these athletes seek such treatments. The most important thing for an athlete is performance. Elite athletes handle pain much better than the average person. They've spent a lifetime playing at a high level. What they cannot accept is a decline in performance. They will pay for the treatments that can help them return to the level of play experienced prior to the injury. Mainstream treatments have not served that purpose.

Pain Relief Is Important. Performance Is Critical

This is why regenerative stem cell treatments started to be used for sports injuries. Pain relief is important. But performance is critical. This means the treatment should cause more benefit than harm. Local tissues have to be preserved so they can regenerate and grow. They should not be removed from the body. This can further weaken the injury site.

Most sports injuries can be managed when properly diagnosed first. Rest, simple physical therapy, and/or well-performed regenerative stem cell therapy may be all that's needed to help people stay active and continue to do the things they love. One great joy in life is the ability to stay active.

Unfortunately, the more active we are, the more wear and tear there is. This creates a greater risk of injury. While staying active is important, wear and tear shouldn't cause you to stop the activities you enjoy. The reverse is what happens most often. Athletes are often advised to slow down or even stop their activities. Slowly the athletes become withdrawn and depressed. Stem cells have shown tremendous benefits to heal many sports injuries, even alleviating pain and arthritis.

Your Own Cells Can Regenerate

The goal of stem cell treatment is to regenerate and repair. And as noted before, your own cells can be the safest source. Heal the injury by replacing damaged cells with native cells. No surgery or other treatments can claim the regeneration process. Stem cell therapy is the only treatment that will actually regenerate tissue. This means you won't replace damaged tissue with scar tissue. This process creates actual tissue.

The stem cell therapy process has a significant impact on not only healing the injury but also keeping you pain-free. You will be able to perform the activities you love. It's not important how long you have been suffering from pain. It's not even important whether your pain is moderate or severe. If your pain is significant enough to limit the activities you love, stem cells may help.

Regenerative stem cell therapy using PRP as well as mesenchymal stem cell injections can help athletes recover quickly without significant downtime. Obviously, the effectiveness of the treatment depends on the protocol used. To repeat a point we've made before, not all stem cell treatments are the same. The manner in which the treatment is applied can be very different. The risks can vary also. Be careful before you choose a particular kind of stem cell treatment.

One important distinction is what treatment you're getting. And for what purpose. Platelet-rich plasma by itself is a potent anti-inflammatory. It can be done at the site of the injury. However, when you're dealing with an actual tear, damage, and tissue loss, you need a large number of your own mesenchymal stem cells in order to have a successful outcome. PRP by itself isn't enough to complete the entire repair process. Sometimes folks making recommendations to athletes do not understand the subtle differences between the different kinds of cells and their applications. The following questions need to be answered before your stem cell treatment is performed:

- What is the source of the stem cells being used?
- What are the risks involved with the use of stem cells?
- How many live stem cells will be administered?
- How will the stem cells be delivered to the site of your injury?
- How many treatments will you need for complete healing to take place?
- What is the rehab plan for your recovery phase following the treatment?
- When will you be back playing your sports?

It can get extremely frustrating. You often hear athletic superstar success stories. On the other hand, you hear mixed reports about stem cell treatment success. Some athletes wait for months hoping to heal. Later they are told to get surgery. Valuable time can be lost.

It's important to understand that the term "stem cell treatment" means nothing in relation to a specific treatment. Lack of standardization is a big concern. Treatment outcomes, complications, and natural courses cannot be compared. This is because treatment protocols may have varied. Currently, there are no apples-to-apples comparisons. Every treatment can be different and unique depending on the condition. Mainstream doctors often don't understand the field of stem cells. The physicians you should see are those who specialize in stem cells.

Stem cells are not a solution for every sports injury. The science isn't there yet. But an insufficient treatment, or one that's not performed correctly, won't get results. A decision between surgery and any other form of treatment should be made in the beginning. This should start with a proper diagnosis of the extent of your injury.

Stem Cells After Surgery

Another area to look into is the role of stem cells after surgery. Since stem cells by nature are anti-inflammatory, they can help clear up inflammation caused by surgery. They can also play a significant role after surgery in minimizing scar tissue formation. Surgery focuses on mechanically fixing problems—taking stitches where there's a tear or removing a part of the damaged tissue. Stem cells can help natural tissue regrow, improving outcomes. Surgery may also be unable to address all the damage associated with an injury. Targeted stem cell injection can help in addressing some of those areas where no other clear solution exists.

Every Athlete Should Consider Stem Cell Therapy

Every athlete should look into these options before deciding on the best course of treatment. Every organ in your body is full of stem cells. They can serve as a source of your own treatment. The most commonly used sources are your own fat, muscle, bone marrow, and blood. Removing some of these tissues does not affect your body in any way, and these tissues can all be safely collected. All these tissues have millions of stem cells. These cells can be isolated and utilized to help repair damage in your joints, cartilage, meniscus, bone, muscles, and ligaments. These cells come from the same family that forms these structures. Unlike stem cell treatments involving other organs, no laboratory manipulation is required.

Different stem cell sources are being evaluated. Your own stem cells are the ones best suited to heal without the risk of introducing anything foreign into your body. Nature has prepackaged the ability to heal yourself. What price would you put on that kind of freedom and ability to do things you love?

Taking Care of Your Body

As an athlete, you are bombarded with nutritional supplements and all kinds of advice. You probably know the importance of taking care of your body. You know how to do the right thing. However, every natural supplement that comes in a bottle is not natural. Do not believe it. Do not trust it. Your body is your biggest pharmacy. Learn to harness the power of your own body. Doing too much is not going to be helpful. Stick to the fundamentals. These are more important than anything flashy out there.

The fundamentals are focused on hydration and a balanced diet. It really doesn't matter whether you have tap, bottled, sparkling, or pH-balanced water; you need pure, simple hydration. Getting a gallon of water into your body every day keeps your cells healthy and happy. The same goes for food. Look for more natural sources. Whether you eat vegetables, fish, or meat products, eat from natural sources rather than packaged processed food.

Getting enough sleep is another important aspect of healing. Though the amount of time one sleeps is variable, about six to eight hours is considered essential. It's also important to know the difference between icing and heating. It is good to ice an acute injury. It can minimize bleeding. Cold from ice causes blood vessels in the applied area to shut down. This is the same reason why icing is recommended after surgery. However, after the acute phase is over, heat does best in order for your injury to heal.

Heat opens up blood vessels and improves flow to the local area. Nutrition has to get down to the cells in the area of injury. You need more blood in that area. The heat helps generate more blood flow. One of the cheapest investments you can make is buying a decent heating pad. This is one that can deliver high-intensity consistent heat. Why? Because your body is taking a daily hit. Your joints, muscles, and ligaments are getting inflamed. Waiting for the pain to get worse is not good. Daily multiple applications of heat to the area that is hurting or sore is the best thing you can do. This will promote local regeneration and repair.

As you regenerate and repair the injury, the next question is whether the rehab is structured properly and specifically to your individual condition. During the rehab phase, no matter what the treatment, it is very important to address what caused the injury in the first place. Look at your body. Evaluate the mechanics involved in the injury. Pay attention to the pre-injury routine and sequence of events. Look at the external factors that contributed. These are all important. You don't want to repeat those contributing factors and reinjure yourself.

Next, focus on your whole body. So much attention during rehab is placed on the injured site. The injury's connection to other parts of the body is ignored. You're not made of concrete and steel. Your body is one whole unified structure. Unless your whole body is in sync, you are likely to suffer another injury. It is not uncommon to see an athlete injure a knee after coming back from an ankle injury or vice versa. Therefore, it is extremely important for you to educate yourself and be an active participant in designing your rehab.

KEY TAKEAWAYS

1. Injury prevention is better than a cure. Cross-train in multiple sports.

2. "No pain, no gain" is *false*. Pain is the body's way of telling you to stop. Find out the reason for your pain before you continue. Get the right diagnosis.

3. Rest and recovery are critical to performance. Your goal is to perform, not just play. Respect your body.

4. Your own stem cells can heal you. It's a new tool. Look for a physician who specializes in stem cells. Understand your treatment.

5. Unfortunately, your sports organization's training staff and team physicians may not always have your best interest. Seek opinions outside your immediate circle.

CHAPTER 8

Stem Cells
and Your Sex Life

A healthy sex life ties into your physical, mental, spiritual,
and emotional well-being.

Letting Go of the Pills

CASE STUDY: DANIEL

At 22, Daniel noticed an inability to maintain an erection. Even
during masturbation, his penis would soften quickly. He was not
sure what the problem was. He thought binging on porn when he
was younger was the culprit. He felt shame and guilt. He couldn't
even discuss it with anyone. He feared becoming the butt of jokes.

Daniel was otherwise healthy and participated in sports regularly. He had a few stress factors complicating his life outside sex.
He started to take the popular pills. But they didn't work. He was

disgusted every time he took them. The side effect was nausea, which he couldn't tolerate. The expectation that he was too young for medication caused even more stress. He avoided sex with his girlfriend. The relationship ended soon after. The campus doctor referred him to a clinical psychologist. Sean was reluctant to discuss anything. He had a wonderful childhood. His parents were happily married and supportive. He had no other issues until this occurred.

Daniel was referred to a urologist. He underwent a battery of tests, including all the basics: blood work, hormone level tests, and even blood flow studies to and from the penis. Sean was diagnosed with vein leakage in his penis. A simple outpatient surgical procedure could be the cure. Sean was looking forward to it. He was excited to finally have a diagnosis and a suggested cure. With the fix he would gain freedom. Sean was even relieved he could discuss his condition with others for the first time without guilt.

CASE STUDY: **MEGAN**

Megan was a 45-year-old housewife and proud mother of three. Her husband was an attorney. Over the past year, she noticed an intense deep pelvic pain during and immediately after sexual intercourse. Initially, she brushed it off as related to a dietary product. She tried taking anti-inflammatories. Months passed. The pain became persistent. She sought an evaluation from her gynecologist. He didn't find any abnormalities during a clinical exam. Nonetheless, an ultrasound of her pelvis was recommended. The exam was normal. The pain became even more intense. At this point, she avoided sex.

Because she was feeling extremely distressed, her gynecologist recommended a psychologist. Megan felt the pain and didn't think it was in her head. The psychologist spent hours asking about her past. He was focused on sexual abuse. Her sex life had always been satisfying. She had a flourishing career as a teacher until she took a break to become a mom. Megan could not see any connection. The psychologist concluded that her subconscious was the cause. She was actually suffering from depression.

Megan was referred to a med-prescribing psychiatrist. On her first visit, he recommended antidepressants. She was told the stress of raising kids and being confined to the house could be contributing to her symptoms.

Clearly nothing physically was found in any of the tests. The expert opinion was that the cause was psychological, not physical. A year had passed. Though not a big fan of medications, Megan decided to try antidepressants. After three more months, the pain was still there. At this point, she stopped all sexual activity with her husband. Her condition also put a strain on their marriage. She saw more gynecologists to find a solution. Each visit led nowhere, leaving her dejected. The doctors wouldn't believe her symptoms.

Another two years passed. Her constant worry was now taking a physical toll—Megan had lost 35 pounds. On a local morning TV show, a young doctor spoke about a condition known to cause pain during and after intercourse. Pelvic congestion syndrome caused the size of the pelvic vein to increase along with the pooling of blood within the veins. This happened during or immediately after physical activity, especially sexual intercourse. The veins in the pelvis around the uterus and ovaries were affected. The doctor mentioned that pelvic congestion syndrome is an often-missed condition. Even an ultrasound would be insufficient to diagnose it. This was music to Megan's ears. After almost five years of agony and misery and wasted time with gynecologists, psychologists, and psychiatrists, she finally had hope. The scores of medications she was taking would only do more harm. Her marriage was falling apart, although she and her husband were still together for the sake of the kids. She sought consultation with the new doctor. Megan finally had an answer to her sexual dysfunction.

Sexual Dysfunction: Is It Physical or Mental?

The cases of Daniel and Megan highlight that sexual dysfunction is not always psychological. Though often labeled as purely psychological, a physical cause must be ruled out first. So many conditions involving the penis in men and the pelvis in women are missed. Nowhere else in medicine are patients so quickly diagnosed as having mental problems as when they seek help for a sex-related disorder. This is especially true for women and young males.

The good news is that most cases of sexual dysfunction have a well-defined cause and can be treated. Clearly there are some psychological causes leading to sexual dysfunction. However, most of the time it is the other way around. When patients don't find the right diagnosis or treatment for their sexual dysfunction, they are more likely to feel depressed and frustrated. This sets up a cycle of both physical and psychological consequences.

Sexual Dysfunction

Sexual dysfunction constitutes major problems. Globally, 300 million men experience difficulty getting or maintaining an erection, a condition known as erectile dysfunction, or ED. Besides

ED, men suffer from premature ejaculation, no ejaculation, and loss of interest in sex (low libido).

The condition is more complex in women. The spectrum of sexual dysfunction in women may involve different phases of sexual activity. These include low sexual desire, aversion to sexual contact, inadequate vaginal lubrication, inability to orgasm, and pain during sexual intercourse. These symptoms, despite the women's desire or wish to engage in sexual activity, constitute female sexual dysfunction. One-third of women under 50 and a half above 50 have experienced sexual dysfunction.

Sexual Dysfunction Causes

Common causes of dysfunction are poor blood flow (commonly seen in middle age) and poor circulation. A lack of adequate blood flow adds a physical component to the problem. As we age, blood vessels become narrower and harder. This makes it difficult for adequate blood flow to reach the sex organs for proper functioning. One in four men under the age of 40 have ED. In younger men, the onset of ED may be a sign of impending heart disease. Underlying obesity, diabetes, and high blood pressure can contribute to sexual dysfunction. Substance abuse, including smoking and alcoholism, is another major cause. Hormone imbalances such as lack of testosterone, estrogen, thyroid, and other hormones can contribute.

Psychological issues such as depression, negative body image, emotional neglect, eating disorders, stress, anxiety, and sexual abuse can certainly play a role. Cultural perceptions, the way sexual issues were addressed during youth, and parental and family stigmas can all shape attitudes toward sex.

Finally, there are medications that can decrease libido, including antidepressants, medicines for high blood pressure, and heartburn medications. Also, be careful of so-called natural supplements. You can never be sure of their ingredients. Don't be fooled by the labels. While the cause can be psychological, underlying physical factors cannot be ignored.

Extremely important in managing sexual dysfunction is to first have a detailed evaluation of the patient's history and a thorough physical examination. Men with a psychogenic basis tend to maintain their early-morning erections as well as during masturbation. This could be important in distinguishing the causes of ED.

A lot of doctors do not know how to treat sexual dysfunction. They may not take your symptoms seriously. Physical and psychological components get intermixed. It becomes a mess after a while. Ultrasound evaluation of pelvic/penile blood flow provides a good idea about the adequacy of circulation or any abnormalities related to the flow of blood. Psychological evaluation is always an important step in managing sexual dysfunction. Stress, anxiety, and depression can all lead to performance anxiety, irrespective of any other underlying cause.

Sex Med Effects

CASE STUDY: **GEORGE**

George, a 49-year-old bank executive, was excited about the weekend. He and his girlfriend planned on spending time at an island resort. Even though George was healthy, the stress of work sometimes could interfere with his daily life. His friend recommended that George take a famous blue pill so that he could really enjoy his time on the island.

One evening in the middle of intercourse, George's whole body went limp. He fell unconscious in the arms of his girlfriend. She had no clue what happened. She noticed that George took a blue pill earlier that evening. She immediately called the front desk to call the EMS. When the squad arrived, George was short of breath and unconscious. He was unresponsive to any stimuli. One of the paramedics put a tube down George's throat to maintain breathing. The island had no more than a basic medical clinic. George was airlifted by helicopter to the closest tertiary-level medical center. He was lucky to receive prompt help given that he had been on an island.

Upon his arrival, a battery of tests was performed. Among those was a CT scan showing a large amount of blood in his brain. George had bleeding during sexual intercourse. He would undergo more testing and likely have a prolonged recovery.

Studies have shown that commonly prescribed sex-stimulating medications can cause a sudden increase in blood pressure. These can lead to heart attacks, bleeding in the brain, and buildup of fluid in the lungs.

The TV Cure

Current treatments of sexual dysfunction are focused on medications like the famous "blue pill." There are ads on TV for pills, hormone shots, and even creams. Pills can be taken orally or through placement in the urethra (the opening from where you pee). Chemical penile injections just prior to sexual activity offer another method. In the short run, these treatments work. Common side effects of these remedies include headaches, flushing face, upset stomach, and impaired vision. More rare but serious side effects are high blood pressure, chest pain, heart attack, stroke, blindness, loss of hearing, and priapism (an erection lasting for longer than four hours). Some patients opt for vacuum devices and implants. Surgical implants come with their own risks and are usually not reversible. Think extremely hard (no pun intended) before you opt for one. Treatments are also focused on psychotherapy with the aid of a sex therapist. Behavioral interventions may be helpful in certain cases. Obviously, a proper diagnosis is key to deciding on the right treatment option for you. Getting down to the root cause along with understanding the complete dynamics of the sexual dysfunction in your individual case is key to a cure.

ED Is a Symptom, Not a Diagnosis

CASE STUDY: ANDY

Andy is a 38-year-old truck driver hauling big semis. He works for a multinational company and drives across the country. He has noticed decreased erections for the past nine months. They have progressively gone weaker. It has gotten to a point where he's unable to initiate an erection. This has started to impact his married life. His wife is suspicious since Andy spends so much time on the road. She has asked him if he's sleeping with other women or having an affair.

Andy feels very frustrated. His doctor brushed Andy's symptoms aside as stress and fatigue from work. Andy was given a few pills. He took them, but he didn't see any results. They also upset his stomach and gave him an uneasy feeling in his chest. On follow-up with his doctor, Andy was referred to a psychotherapist for evaluation. During the third session at the psychotherapist's office, it was becoming more and more clear that Andy didn't have any psychological issues. Nor did he have any past or family history of psychological problems. But he did tell his psychologist that he may no longer drive trucks. This was due to cramping pain in his buttocks. Andy attributed that to the long hours of sitting and driving. His psychologist wondered when the buttock pain had started. It was about the same time as the difficulty with his erections. His psychologist advised Andy he should have a complete physical examination. It had been several years since he had a complete workup.

Andy subsequently underwent a physical as well as blood work. Most of his labs turned out to be normal. However, during his physical exam, the doctor noted some loss of hair on his legs and feet. His legs also felt a little cooler, and the arterial pulse in his groin was weak. Andy was referred to a vascular specialist. He underwent a CTA scan to study the blood vessels in his abdomen and his pelvis. A blockage was found in his arteries, and this was compromising blood flow to his penis. Andy's condition even has a name; it is called "Leriche syndrome." Andy underwent a revascularization procedure to open up the blocked artery. This restored blood flow to his penis. Andy started having full erections just as he used to.

Again, this case highlights how erectile dysfunction has several physical causes. Unfortunately, a lot of men risk dangerous medications. They waste time visiting psychiatrists and taking medications for depression due to their ED. Remember ED is a symptom, not a diagnosis. Always look for a cause.

Regeneration and Circulation

CASE STUDY: **JAMES**

James is 50 years old. He is an attorney with a successful practice and has raised two wonderful boys with his wife, Nelly. About three years ago, the boys transitioned from high school to college. Before their biological clock ran out, the couple decided to have another child. They wisely made time for more sexual activity. But soon they started to notice something was wrong. James was not able to maintain an erection. Soon it progressed to the point where it was difficult even getting one. Initially, he thought it was due to fatigue from work. James otherwise had led a pretty healthy life.

James sought the advice of his primary care physician. Reassuringly, James was told not to worry; it would soon pass. He started to cut down his workload. Six months later, there was no sign of improvement. Feeling even more anxious and embarrassed, James requested that his primary care doc refer him to a urologist. After a brief examination, the urologist recommended a course of pills designed to improve blood flow to his penis. After three months, James did not notice any significant improvement. He was also concerned about the side effects of these chemicals. His urologist also suggested a penile implant. James could not wrap his head around this, especially considering an implant would be permanent.

Dejected, James looked for a more natural, holistic option. He started researching and talking to friends about his experience with erectile dysfunction. James came across case reports describing stem cell treatments. Curious, James decided to further explore this option. He was educated enough to avoid falling for some clinic solely based on advertising. He sought the advice of a physician specializing in regenerative treatments. He wanted a doctor with stem cell experience.

James was informed that stem cells are extremely new and not the holy grail. There is also little evidence to support their use. James had the opportunity to ask several questions and yet never felt pressured. What got James interested was the science behind stem cells. He was surprised to find out that stem cells have capabilities to treat inflammation. They can help develop new blood vessels and also replace damaged and old cells. From a scientific point of view, this did make sense. Especially if his own stem cells could be used, the risk would be minimal.

His physician emphasized that there is a subset of patients, for yet unknown reasons, who do not respond to stem cell treatments. The same applies to any treatment, individual responses vary due to our different genetic and environmental makeup. James had himself not responded well to the popular blue pill that everybody swears by. With stem cell treatment having very few side effects, James opted for the stem cell approach. However, it was important to James that the treatment be as natural as possible, avoiding foreign chemicals.

He was fully aware it was experimental and may not work. Other options his urologist recommended weren't appealing. The stem cells were delivered by injections at strategic points on James's penis. He had a total of three treatments over a period of six months. Each time he noticed an improvement in the quality of his erections. Nelly soon got pregnant, and the couple had their third child. Two years after his stem cell treatments, James and Nelly enjoy as much sex as the infant permits.

Stem cells promote blood flow by decreasing inflammation and creating new blood vessels. When no other physical cause is found, patients often rely on medications possessing serious side effects. A better and safer alternative would be the application of platelet-rich plasma and mesenchymal stem cells in sexual dysfunction. Several case reports have been published that detail successful treatments using these methods. More studies are needed to clearly distinguish real gains from placebo effects. Your own mesenchymal stem cells derived from your own body have proved to be largely safe. Given the safety of stem cells compared with sexual dysfunction pills, the regenerative alternative seems a choice worth exploring.

Complementary Treatments

Cures such as shock wave therapy are gaining popularity in the United States. Even though these kinds of treatments have been around Europe for years, there are no robust studies of them. The devices that produce shock waves work by inducing a low-level trauma to stimulate blood vessel flow in sexual organs. Some advocates use the devices in conjunction with stem cell treatments. More research is required to prove both the extent and duration of their effectiveness.

Boost Your Sexual Performance

"Your body follows your mind" could not be truer when it comes to sexual health. It's all about either the mind or the blood flow. You can optimize your health by doing some basic things:

- One of the best is to gather the courage to discuss any problems with your partner. The only caveat is whether the partner is a cause of the problem! A lot of sexual problems become worse because of people hiding their dysfunction from their partners. Your partner won't feel trusted if you don't open up. This starts a vicious cycle. Also, the stress generated from holding on to a sexual issue further complicates the problem. There is no reason to feel guilty or ashamed. Sharing your problems with your partner will only make you more comfortable.

- Relax your mind. Meditation works as well as walking barefoot on the beach or listening to music. Do whatever will help you get into a state of peace and calm. Make it part of your daily routine.

- Have a good sleep schedule. This is important to maintaining enough energy to perform sexually. You need the stamina and peace of mind to sustain a good performance!

- Maintain your hydration, and watch your sugar intake and weight. Pomegranate juice and walnuts both have been shown to promote nitric oxide formation. Nitric oxide is a wonderful compound that opens up blood vessels and improves circulation. As we age, nitric oxide production goes down. Other natural sources that can help promote nitric oxide buildup include beets, garlic, raw cacao, and spinach. Pomegranate fruit has been shown to be safe even for diabetics. It can actually improve glucose metabolism over a period of time.

- The most effective thing you can do for great sex is to consistently exercise. It is not the intensity but the consistency that is important. Is it part of your daily routine right now? Exercise helps build stamina, improves cardiovascular health, and develops sustained endurance. Exercise involving lifting is one of the best ways to boost your sex hormone production. Exercise reduces stress and elevates mood.

As you can see, there are so many natural ways to improve sexual performance. Your own stem cells are an emerging tool that can help. But your own stem cells will not be effective if you aren't healthy and strong. Each of these recommendations will promote flow. It is amazing just how beneficial these various tools can be. Make them a part of your daily life. Healthy sex is an important component of our lives. We should harness our inner energies by cultivating a healthy mind and body. It's a privilege. Don't take it for granted.

KEY TAKEAWAYS

1. Ensure a proper diagnosis. Seek a thorough evaluation. Physical causes are easily curable provided you first get a proper diagnosis. Don't buy into the "psychological-only" reasoning.
2. Share your problem with your partner. Do not feel ashamed or guilty.
3. Stay away from pills, other drugs, and chemical injections.
4. Take care of your body. Improve blood flow with daily exercise and pomegranates.
5. Consider whether your own stem cells can help. Talk with an expert.
6. Keep your mind calm. Meditate, relax, and stay in the moment.

CHAPTER 9

Stem Cells and
Your Heart and Lungs

The key to improving longevity . . .

Stem Cells and Your Heart

Dr. Michael E. DeBakey, the world-famous heart surgeon of the 20th century, performed a record number of surgeries due to clogged arteries. In the days before his death, Dr. DeBakey became convinced that arterial blockages were due to inflammation in the artery walls.

For decades, physicians have focused on cholesterol as the cause of clogged arteries. But now research has shown that cholesterol will stick to the walls of arteries when inflamed. If there is no inflammation, cholesterol will not stick. Several studies have focused on the connection between inflammation and arterial blockage. Several more studies have looked at the exact pathways and cells involved. Research continues to further validate this connection.

Current treatments for arterial blockage consist of medications to decrease cholesterol levels, diet, and lifestyle modifications. When the blockage is severe, therapies such as artery bypass surgery (creating a side channel across the blockage), angioplasty (balloon dilation), and/or stenting (placing a metal scaffold) are done to keep the artery stretched open.

None Address the Blockages

As you can imagine, not bypass surgery, or angioplasty, or stenting addresses the cause of the blockage. This explains, over time, why bypass channels and metal stents also develop blockages. If we can figure out the exact inflammatory pathways that lead to inflammation in the walls of blood vessels, the arterial blockage may be decreased or even eliminated. Stem cells can play a tremendous role in minimizing the risk of these kinds of blockages. There is already preliminary research in the application of stem cells to help treat inflammation in arterial walls.

Stem Cells and Heart Failure

CASE STUDY: **MR. KRAFT**

Mr. Kraft, a businessman in his 70s, worked very hard at building a successful food and catering business. Over the past 10 years, he's dealt with the symptoms of clogged arteries in his heart. Angiography revealed significant multiple blockages. He was not considered a candidate for bypass surgery. Mr. Kraft made significant lifestyle changes in response. He still can't walk long distances without experiencing chest pain. Despite medication, there has not been much clinical improvement. Recent tests have shown a decline in his heart function. The ability of his heart to pump blood is diminishing. His condition has limited his social activities. Depression has followed. His cardiologist could recommend no effective therapy. Mr. Kraft wouldn't accept his sentence of a slow death. Instead, he decided to research stem cell therapy.

After researching the different types and sources of stem cells, Mr. Kraft opted to use his own. After a harvesting procedure and processing, his own stem cells were delivered through a tiny tube placed in his heart. Mr. Kraft experienced no complications. In the next few weeks, Mr. Kraft noticed less chest pain. He is now able to visit the country club once a week. Mr. Kraft was also advised that he might need additional stem cell treatments. That would depend on his progress.

Another area of potential stem cell application is preventing or minimizing heart failure. Heart failure is a common endpoint of heart attacks, coronary artery disease, and high blood pressure—especially when complicated by diabetes.

After a heart attack, there is damage to the heart muscle due to lack of blood supply (which in turn is due to underlying arterial blockage). The damaged heart muscle is usually replaced by scar tissue. This tissue does not have the same function as cardiac muscles, which contract and relax as they pump. In other words, the scarred portion of the heart is not able to contribute to overall functioning. This is how heart failure sets in. As there is more severe repeated damage, the heart becomes weaker.

The heart muscle function eventually diminishes to the extent that it can no longer pump blood to the rest of the body. This ultimately leads to death. This scenario is further complicated due to the heart muscle's poor regenerative capacity.

A heart transplant is not easy either. Not only is it difficult to find a donor's heart, but the burden of major surgery is also often too much to bear. The risk of rejection and the side effects from medication can make life miserable. There are some interim solutions such as an LVAD (left ventricular assist device). This device is like an artificial pump that takes over part of the heart's pumping action. But none of these solutions will preserve, repair, or regenerate your heart.

How Stem Cells Work in the Heart

Research today strives to better understand how stem cells may work in your heart. The goal is to replace scar tissue with live new heart cells that provide the same functionality as other live heart cells. Heart cells, unlike other cells in our body, have very poor regenerative capacity. The heart has fewer stem cells in comparison with other organs. The heart is more like the brain. Both lack the ability to self-repair.

Initially, most of the focus was on embryonic stem cells. They have the capability of growing into any kind of cell. But the direction of therapy over the last 10 years has shifted toward one's own stem cells. Our own stem cells are safest. Still, as we age, they may show some decline in numbers. Their potency may also be reduced.

The next question is, How can we maximize the potential of our cells? Unlike healing cartilage or a meniscus in your knee, heart repair is going to need a lot more stem cells. Also, mesenchymal (fat) stem cells from our body make the repair process much easier and do not require any artificial cell programming. In healing the heart muscle, stem cells have to be specialized enough to replace scar tissue and grow into heart cells.

One way of increasing the number of cells is to take one's own stem cells and multiply them in a laboratory. This can provide a large number of stem cells. This will also eliminate the need to undergo another harvesting procedure. Your own stem cells can be stored, and so multiple treatments may become easier. Within stem cells, there are a variety of cells possessing their own specific functions. The goal is to find out which particular cells, within the population of your own stem cells, promise the greatest chance of heart repair. Another avenue may be to collect your own heart cells from an undamaged area; these cells can then be grown into heart cells in the laboratory.

Two other questions to consider are: Can older people use stem cells donated by younger, healthier folks, and does this provide any advantage? These questions still need to be answered.

Regardless of the sources (embryonic, foreign, or your own adult stem cells), stem cells have shown anti-inflammatory, immune-modulatory (the ability to calm bad cells that attack your own body), and neovascularization (the ability to form new blood vessels) capabilities. Stem cells also release important growth factors, proteins, and compounds that can help regeneration and repair.

Despite all this, the exact mechanism of repair and regeneration in the heart and vascular system is still up for debate. How many stem cells will be needed for repair? How often will the treatments need to be repeated to maximize gains? These are still open questions.

Finally, how are stem cells going to be delivered into the heart? Are they supposed to be introduced by intravenous infusion? Do they have to be delivered via the arteries, intra-arterially through vessels supplying blood to the heart? Intra-arterial delivery of stem cells may limit the extent of damage to the heart muscle. Should stem cells be injected directly into the scarred or dead muscle area of the heart? These questions are still unanswered. Finally, it comes down to which of these methods would benefit the patient most. Stem cells from each individual can show a different ability to grow. As effective as stem cells are, there is a small group of patients who may not respond. Everyone's capacity to heal and grow is different. There could be several reasons. Your general health, environment, and genetic makeup are all factors. All of these affect regeneration and repair.

Nitric Oxide and Blood Flow

One important molecule is nitric oxide (NO). While it's a toxic gas in the atmosphere, it's produced in small quantities in our body. It has shown tremendous benefits. NO has the ability to relax and open up blood vessels. This action improves blood flow to all organ systems. Nitric oxide has shown to be a major player in patients with high blood pressure, heart disease, memory loss, and erectile dysfunction. Besides improving blood flow, it has anti-inflammatory and antioxidant properties. As we age, less and less nitric oxide is produced in the body. Also, the body's signaling pathways (the ability of cells to communicate with each other) may diminish with age. There are several ways to boost nitrous oxide efficiency. Natural sources that can help promote NO buildup are pomegranates, beets, garlic, raw cacao, spinach, and walnuts.

A word about pomegranates: Pomegranate fruit has been extensively studied. Its benefits are most pronounced in circulation and blood flow. Pomegranates are particularly safe in patients with diabetes. Besides improving blood flow, it helps lower blood pressure and decreases bad cholesterol. The benefits of pomegranates on the heart and circulation are so profound that one can safely say, "A pomegranate a day keeps the cardiologist away."

There is tremendous potential for stem cells to help with repair and regeneration of the heart muscle. We are now understanding the capability of stem cells in the heart. We are also getting close to finding the best methods of stem cell heart repair. More clinical trials and data are needed to document improvements. If you or your loved one is considering stem cell treatments, inquire about clinical trials and studies using stem cell treatments for heart failure and associated conditions. Understand the role of stem cells in your situation and the process involved. One of the best things you can do prior to stem cell therapy is to take care of your body. Your blood flow starts from your heart and spreads (through the vascular system) to the rest of your body. A healthy heart and vascular system are critical to proper functioning and enjoyment of your daily life.

Stem Cells and Lungs

CASE STUDY: **JANICE**

Janice was a healthy teenager. Just before going to college, she noticed she was having spells of coughing after exercise. She ignored the spells, attributing them to intense workouts. For relief, she used a variety of cough syrups. One day after jogging, she suddenly started to gasp for air and felt short of breath. She was diagnosed with asthma. From that day on, her life changed.

Now 48, Janice is on steroids and nebulizer treatments. She has been hospitalized multiple times, especially during flu season, contracting many respiratory infections. Janice has been disabled multiple times, impacting her career. Her rescue nebulizer is always at her side. Long flights can be difficult because of the pressure and altitude. She plans all her activities around asthma symptom prevention. Janice has tried every new drug and treatment on the market, desperate to find relief.

There are several lung disorders: asthma, COPD, emphysema, pulmonary fibrosis, interstitial lung disease, pulmonary artery hypertension, and cystic fibrosis. There are even more congenital conditions that can become life-threatening with no available cure. The majority of these conditions start with an acute phase. Soon after, they become chronic. In time, they lead to a loss of lung tissue. Most current treatments are based on symptom control. Medications are merely a stop-gap and do not prevent the loss of lung tissue. In some cases, lung transplantation is recommended. However, because of a shortage of donors, there is generally a long wait. In addition, there is a risk of rejection and the need for medicines that provide lifelong immunosuppression. These become significant downsides. This is one area in which a tremendous amount of research is needed. What are the right types of stem cells most likely to develop into lung cells?

Lung Disease and Inflammation

The majority of lung diseases, especially the common ones, are no different from those we see in other organ systems. They all can become inflamed. On the cellular level, inflammation can cause local structural changes. These changes manifest as symptoms and disease processes.

In asthma, there is a narrowing of the airway due to inflammation in the wall lining. These airways are how we get air in and out of our lungs. Any narrowing can cause shortness of breath, often resulting in a wheezing sound.

Interstitial lung disease is a condition where there is extensive inflammation in the lining supporting lung cells. This progresses to a point where there isn't a healthy gas exchange. The body gets deprived of adequate oxygen. The cells gradually lose their ability to function.

PRP derived from the patients' own blood has been used with promising outcomes. Often these patients don't respond to mainline drug treatments. However, no stem cell lung treatment protocols currently exist. Even using your own mesenchymal (fat) stem cells, clinicians are still learning how lung cell regeneration happens. Your own mesenchymal stem cells (MSCs) do provide anti-inflammatory benefits. But they may not last long enough in the lungs. In order to achieve long-lasting results, these stem cells need to be programmed to grow into lung tissue. Mature adult cells can't do that. Baby cells or modified programmed adult cells have promise but need to be explored. Your own adult MSCs also hold promise and are safest. They certainly will need to be programmed to develop into lung cells. A further question is, How can stem cells be best administered in the lungs? While intravenous administration filters cells in the lungs (cells may get trapped in the tiny blood vessels), all may not stay there. Inhalation and direct implantation are other potential routes. But none have been studied in detail. How many cells and how many treatments will be needed is also largely unknown.

Repair of Lung Cells

Simply put, we do not have enough information or the right kind of stem cells available commercially to consider lung stem cell treatment as a routine valid option. Stem cells can be effective if they demonstrate the capability of actually regenerating and growing new lung cells. There has been proof of regeneration in animal studies. Applying the treatment used in the studies to humans is the next step. Be careful of advertised stem cell treatments for lung conditions. No scientific basis exists yet. Until we find the right stem cell therapy to heal your lungs, maintaining a healthy lifestyle is your best bet. Follow instructions from your pulmonologist, and keep exploring newer treatment options.

KEY TAKEAWAYS

1. Stem cells for heart research are now more advanced; we are getting closer to treatments.
2. Stem cells for lungs are at the beginning stages, and protocols have not been clearly defined.
3. Do not give up on your doctor's traditional recommendations unless you clearly understand what role stem cells will play in your individual case.
4. Maintain a healthy body, and don't forget the pomegranate for maintaining strong blood flow.

CHAPTER 10

Stem Cells and Autoimmune Conditions

Diabetes, Kidney Failure, and Lupus

When your body becomes your enemy . . .

Improving Your Quality of Life

Autoimmune disease happens when your body turns against its own cells. The body normally attacks foreign invaders such as bacteria and viruses. This is called "immunity." When the body loses the ability to distinguish between foreign invaders and its own cells, it becomes autoimmune. This is when the immune system attacks healthy cells. Some of the most common autoimmune diseases are rheumatoid arthritis, systemic lupus erythematosus (or SLE), scleroderma, Graves' disease, type 1 (or juvenile) diabetes, and inflammatory bowel disease. There are several other conditions too.

Autoimmune conditions can be hard to diagnose depending upon which organ system is affected. Most patients have swelling and inflammation of the joints. They have an inability to complete tasks because of extreme fatigue. No matter how much rest, they still feel tired. Fatigue is often accompanied by a low-grade fever. Muscle pain, hair loss, skin rashes, and sores can also occur in autoimmune conditions. The ability to work is greatly affected, and patients often have to rearrange their daily routines.

As their condition progresses, inflammation of the kidneys, lungs, and other organs can occur. Symptoms may go on for several years before a diagnosis is made. What causes your body to become an enemy is unknown. If you have a family history of autoimmune disorders, your risk goes up. There is no prevention. Once set in, the condition will be for life. There is no cure.

Stems Cells and Diabetes

CASE STUDY: **EVELYN**

Evelyn runs her own successful digital marketing company. A typical millennial, she exercises regularly and has been careful about what she eats. She struggled with more headaches over the past few months. She initially attributed these symptoms to overwork and too much computer time. As time went by, the headaches became more frequent and unpredictable. Convinced they were migraines, she went to see a neurologist. Her doctor ordered some basic blood tests, which showed high blood sugar levels. Evelyn was shocked. But more advanced testing confirmed type 1 diabetes.

Evelyn did not fit the profile of a type 1 diabetic, which is usually diagnosed at a much younger age. She was a 42-year-old successful business owner, a loving mom, and a devoted wife trying to make the right decisions. Evelyn soon started receiving insulin injections. The shots were administered three to five times a day. She had to reorganize her schedule. She also had to constantly monitor her blood sugar levels.

The impact of diabetes can be devastating. It can have an emotional, psychological, physical, and even economic impact.

Diabetes is a disease producing extremely high blood sugar levels. This is caused by an inability of the body to provide insulin, a hormone secreted by your pancreas. Insulin regulates your blood sugar level. The lack of insulin production leads to high blood sugar levels. High blood sugar is damaging to cells and leads to organ complications and ultimately premature death.

Two of the most common forms of diabetes are:

- **Type 2 (the most well known).** This type of diabetes normally occurs in adults and is commonly associated with being overweight. It starts off as insulin resistance and turns to insulin deficiency.
- **Type 1.** Diabetes may start early in life, occurring when the body lacks insulin-producing cells. The body produces very little or no insulin from the beginning.

No matter the type, it is important to understand that diabetes is a chronic condition that affects the entire body. It impacts the heart, blood vessels, eyes, and nervous system and also increases the chance of infections. Just as importantly, it decreases the regenerative capacity of the entire body.

The International Diabetes Federation reports more than 4 million people died from diabetes in 2017 and almost half were under 60. Type 2 diabetes is increasing worldwide. Surprisingly, half of diabetics are unaware they have the disease. Most people develop diabetes between the ages of 40 and 59.

Diabetes also has a tremendous social and economic impact. The economic impact is twofold. First, it leads to loss of productivity, and second, the cost of treatment and the healthcare burden from complications is significant.

Diabetes impacts the immediate family, relatives, and caregivers. Dietary modifications and exercise can help. Existing treatments for diabetes focus on insulin replacement and/or medications, all attempting to modify glucose metabolism. Most medications have side effects. Some can be debilitating. Current treatments for diabetes are lifelong and must be followed daily for the rest of your life. These treatments can significantly impact your lifestyle.

Thankfully, stem cells can play an important role in the treatment of diabetes. Stem cell therapy can eliminate the need for daily drugs and insulin shots. But more importantly, cell regeneration can help avoid life-threatening complications.

Currently, there are no established proven stem cell treatment protocols that can be used clinically. Stem cells can help if researchers find a way to regrow insulin-producing cells. To be effective, insulin-producing cells must grow again and help the body produce its own insulin. Until that happens, we cannot expect a cure.

Whether the cell source is foreign (embryonic or birth-related tissue) or autologous (your own cells), source cells will need to be preprogrammed in a laboratory. This will ensure they have the potential to produce insulin when implanted in your body. These cells may be delivered in your pancreas or placed at another site.

CASE STUDY: **SARAH**

Sarah was a healthy 12-year-old who loved playing softball. Over the past few weeks, her mother noticed that her motivation to play was decreasing. Sarah looked extremely tired even after a good night's rest. She seemed very reluctant to go to practice, even though that after-school activity used to be the highlight of her day. Sarah was also losing weight. This concerned her mom, who took Sarah for a checkup. Sarah had high blood sugar and was diagnosed with type 1 diabetes. No one else in her family had the disease. Sarah had to endure multiple hospital and emergency room visits. She was constantly monitoring her blood sugar. Sarah was told diabetes would be with her for the rest of her life. But if she could learn to manage it, she could live normally and do everything a healthy person could do.

Type 1 diabetes is really tough on the patient. It impacts every aspect of life. Patients have to plan everything around keeping control of blood sugar. The real problem with diabetes is that it can affect every organ in your body. If you do not manage diabetes properly, several complications can develop down the road. These complications can take a heavy toll on your health.

One common complication is low blood sugar (hypoglycemia), which can cause a feeling of confusion, dizziness, and even a coma, among other problems. In addition, without insulin, there is an uncontrolled breakdown of fat to provide glucose (diabetic ketoacidosis), which can cause the person to lose consciousness. Other complications include vision loss (diabetic retinopathy); pain, tingling, and numbness in your legs (diabetic neuropathy); and kidney failure.

Complications often lead to hospitalization. More importantly, these complications can decrease your lifespan. There have been several advances in medicine, including continuous glucose monitoring devices and insulin pumps. These advances have made diabetes slightly easier to manage.

Currently there is extensive stem cell research trying to grow insulin-producing cells that can be implanted into the patient's body. This will allow insulin to be delivered naturally. Also, various clinical trials are in progress attempting to define which stem cells will be most effective and how they can be applied to help promote insulin production. However, there is no proven stem cell treatment yet. So beware of falling for most advertised treatments. These are scams. You can waste significant amounts of your time and money on them.

An area of diabetes where stem cells can also play an important role is in managing complications. Wound infection and other inflammatory processes can especially affect the whole body. The risk and severity of infection can be twice as great in patients with diabetes. Pain nerve fibers are heightened in the early stages. Many routine procedures can be a lot more painful for diabetic patients than others. In advanced stages, nerves become damaged and lose sensation. This can lead to injuries and wounds even without the patient feeling them. Similarly, any invasive procedure like surgery can be twice as risky in a patient with diabetes.

Mesenchymal (fat) stem cells harvested from your own body can be helpful. Their anti-inflammatory, immune-modulatory (calm the cells that are destroying your body), and vasculogenic (support growth of new blood vessels) properties can potentially help control the progression of diabetes complications. Multiple treatments may be required. But well-defined protocols don't yet exist. Further research is needed in this area.

As noted earlier in the book, one fruit that has shown to help regulate blood sugar levels in diabetes patients is the pomegranate. Several studies have shown that the sugar inside the pomegranate fruit is not harmful. Unlike other fruits, the pomegranate does not increase blood sugar levels. This fruit possesses antioxidants and other beneficial compounds that can help the body control sugar levels. The pomegranate can also significantly improve blood sugar levels over a period of time. Unfortunately, this fruit can be hard to find in some parts of the world. Also, most commercially sold pomegranate juice is fortified with artificial sugar. Try to find a source that contains pure cold-pressed pomegranate juice without additives. Check your local farmers market; you will be surprised.

There is one positive note about Evelyn and Sarah. Both are now actively engaged in raising funds for diabetes research that explores the use of stem cells. Evelyn is looking forward to the day when she and millions of others can claim their lives back. Sarah is busy applying for college softball scholarships. If you want more information about diabetes, stay connected with the local chapter of the International Diabetes Federation. This worldwide organization provides important resources. Only by networking with patients in similar situations can our lives be improved.

Stem Cells and Kidney Failure

Diabetes can cause kidney failure. Although there are several other causes, half of all patients with kidney failure have diabetes. Once the kidneys fail, dialysis may be the only way to survive unless you are a transplant candidate. Donor kidneys can be hard to find, and you have to be in good general health to be considered. Even if a matched donor kidney is found, the process of transplant involves many toxic medications. These are to prevent your immune system from rejecting the new kidney.

Toxic medications prescribed before and after transplant can cause significant side effects. Even when patients survive major transplant surgery, they often fall victim to the side effects of the medications. Normal kidneys remove toxins and other waste material. After kidneys fail, their functions have to be replaced.

Dialysis is the process of removing waste material and clearing toxins. In order to keep your body clean, dialysis has to be performed three to five times per week. There are two ways of doing dialysis. One is peritoneal dialysis, or PD. A semipermanent plastic tube is placed inside your abdomen. The outer end of the tube is on the surface of your belly. During dialysis, the outer end of the tube is hooked to a portable dialysis machine. A special fluid goes in and out of your belly and through the inside lining. It cleans the body of waste and toxins. Some patients can do this at home while asleep. PD has several advantages. It causes minimum interference in a patient's daily life and activities. Patients can even carry the peritoneal dialysis machine when they travel.

Another method of doing dialysis is directly through blood vessels. This procedure is called "hemodialysis." Two special dialysis needles, one inflow and one outflow, are stuck directly into your blood vessels. One needle draws the blood out of your body. Then the blood runs through a dialysis machine. The other needle puts the clean blood back into your body. A hemodialysis setup is quite elaborate. While hemodialysis can be done at home, most patients use a dialysis center. Hemodialysis is performed every other day of the week. Each dialysis session can last anywhere from two to four hours. This obviously limits and interferes with the patient's daily routine.

Dialysis is never a permanent solution. The reason is that with any kind of dialysis, the big risk is an infection and/or blockage to the flow. Dialysis patients live in constant fear, striving to make sure neither happens. Otherwise, they may not be able to get dialyzed.

CASE STUDY: **MARIA**

Maria had been diagnosed with type 2 diabetes 20 years ago. For the past 7 years, she dealt with renal failure and has endured hemodialysis. Her family friend Tania had a similar condition and had been on hemodialysis for several years. One day Tania had to race to the emergency room. She could not get hemodialysis because her blood vessels became blocked. Tania had no more treatment options left and ultimately died. Maria fears this happening to her. She is no longer a candidate for a transplant. She waited many years for a matched donor, but one could not be found. Now her heart is too weak to tolerate surgery. Maria started to search for alternatives. She was determined to see her grandkids grow up. Maria looked into the potential of stem cells for kidney failure but was not able to find a current treatment. Maria is hoping stem cell research for kidneys can move at a faster pace. She is also looking forward to the day when her kidney failure is not the end of the road.

The application of stem cells for treating kidney failure is at a very preliminary stage. Research is being done using the patient's own mesenchymal stem cells and other cells derived from an embryo. The goal with stem cells would be to develop a kidney in the laboratory that can be used for transplantation. When your own stem cells are used, toxic medications may not be required because the risk of rejection is extremely low.

Another application of stem cells would attempt to revive your failed kidney. Even if a portion could be made to function again, it may reduce or eliminate the need for dialysis. Remember, even though nature has bestowed us with two kidneys, only one is required to do the job. How many stem cells need to be delivered and how many will be required to revive a nonfunctioning kidney is currently unknown.

Still, another method is using mesenchymal stem cells from your own body. These cells would be incorporated into your blood during dialysis before your blood is returned into your body. It is known that stem cells release certain proteins and other compounds that can help heal the kidney and potentially repair damaged areas.

Stem Cells and Lupus

Lupus is another autoimmune disease. Your cells can't identify your own body, and so they attack normal organs. Lupus can affect any organ. It commonly causes damage in the skin, bones, joints, and kidneys.

CASE STUDY: **ISABELLA**

Isabella was a 16-year-old teenager when she started feeling unusually fatigued. She had pain in both hip joints. She visited the family doctor and was told to rest. Her pain was probably just the result of growing bones. A few weeks passed. Yet Isabella felt more pain and had trouble even walking upstairs. Her concerned mother took Isabella to the local children's hospital. Isabella underwent a series of blood tests and extensive evaluation by a rheumatologist. She was also advised to get a kidney biopsy. Due to her symptoms and test results, Isabella was diagnosed with systemic lupus erythematosus.

Little did Isabella know that her nightmare was just beginning. She was given a course of steroids in an attempt to reduce
inflammation. She was popping Ibuprofen, which caused nausea.
Even though Isabella felt some relief, her hip joints continued to be
painful. She started taking stronger medications. One was a chemotherapy agent. These agents are drugs designed to kill cancer
cells. The side effects took a heavy toll on Isabella.

Two years passed since her diagnosis. On a follow-up visit,
the radiographs of her hip joints showed extensive deformity with
partial collapse. Isabella was recommended for hip joint replace-
ments on both sides. The news completely devastated her. Just
coming to terms with the diagnosis was difficult. She tried to modify her lifestyle. This once active, bubbly teenager loved to party.
But now it was impossible. Isabella faced the prospect that her
hips may get replaced with metal joints. She was frustrated and
depressed. Her parents couldn't bear her depression and decided
to learn about other treatments.

Mom and dad saw a TV interview with a young woman also
diagnosed with lupus. The girl had adult stem cell therapy and was
now leading a near-normal life. They brought this to the attention
of Isabella's doctors at the children's hospital. The family was
discouraged and told it would risk Isabella's life. Her doctors at
the time said these types of alternative treatments had no proven
scientific basis.

Isabella's parents decided to visit the stem cells specialist to
get more information and see if the therapy made sense. After
a thorough evaluation of Isabella's case and also her past treatment history, the doctor explained the science behind stem cells.
He discussed the various types of stem cells and their efficacy
in helping Isabella. The first goal was to get some relief from
disabling hip pain. The physician was honest and said stem cell
treatments were in the early stages for lupus.

There was some evidence that adult or one's own stem cells, combined with platelet-rich plasma, could help calm the joint inflammation. This could possibly repair and regenerate the damage in Isabella's hips. But lupus is also a systemic problem. The underlying disease has to be controlled. This was even a bigger question. There were no clear answers. But there was the possibility of relieving Isabella's hip pain. The therapy could be done by using her own cells. A chance for less pain, with no side effects and no toxic reaction, was the only good news Isabella had received since her diagnosis.

Isabella received targeted injections into both her hip joints using cells derived from her own bone marrow and blood. The entire treatment was performed in a single sitting. These cells are full of anti-inflammatory products and promote regeneration by clearing the inflammation. Mesenchymal stem cells also help balance the immune system. Six weeks later, Isabella felt no need to take Ibuprofen, as she no longer needed it for the pain. She was able to walk around high school without support. Four months later, Isabella underwent another round of treatment. One year after her second treatment, this young girl was swimming and bicycling and was able to do most things girls her age do. More importantly, the procedure boosted Isabella's self-esteem. It improved her ability to fight a disease she will have to live with for the rest of her life.

Isabella was lucky to get an early diagnosis. Lupus symptoms are so general and nonspecific, the disease can go undiagnosed for years. The condition itself can go quiet and then flare up periodically. Also, there are several other conditions that may mask the kind of lupus that Isabella has. Misdiagnosis is not uncommon.

Help Is Just Around the Corner

When you are diagnosed with an autoimmune disease, you will need treatment for the rest of your life, and this can be very difficult. It's not uncommon to feel overwhelmed, confused, angry, and even guilty. It's easy to blame oneself. Let's be clear; there is absolutely nothing anyone can do to prevent autoimmune disease. But there are things you can do to control it.

When you're diagnosed with this condition, try to do some research. The internet has tons of information, but much isn't factual. There are a lot of horror stories, and some may cause you unnecessary worry. There is a lot of false advertising too, especially when it comes to stem cells. Educating yourself about a diagnosis is important. Engage with the local foundation or association that advocates on behalf of your condition. Be open with your family and friends about what you are going through. Most will understand and be your strongest advocates. Study different treatment options by reaching out to patients who have a similar condition to yours. Eating healthily, exercising, resting, and keeping stress under control can all be helpful in minimizing the impact of an autoimmune disorder.

Ask your doctor questions about any treatment he or she prescribes. The medications prescribed can be toxic and cause additional damage. Follow your doctor's advice, but do your own research. Start exploring other options. But don't fall for scams. The information you have now will prepare you to ask the right questions and not be taken in by false promises. Reach out to experts in the field.

There are lots of resources available. Take time to arm yourself with knowledge. It is the best way to keep your condition under control. Educating others is ultimately the biggest reward. It will also give you purpose. You will be able to help others. These suggestions will help you stay active in managing your condition. Stem cells, because of their anti-inflammatory properties and their ability to calm your immune system, have tremendous potential in the treatment of autoimmune conditions.

However, there are many unanswered questions. You should explore stem cell treatments that specifically address your condition. Be aware of the role stem cells will play in your individual situation. Have a good idea of the outcome you can expect. Any real stem cell treatment center should be able to answer these questions. And let us emphasize once again, stay away from the con artists and clinics that claim a quick fix.

KEY TAKEAWAYS

1. Understand your autoimmune diagnosis. Learn as much as you can.

2. Network with your local foundation's or association's advocacy group.

3. Don't lose hope. Some days will be more difficult than others. Take care of your body and mind.

4. Remember that help is around the corner. Stem cells have already shown their effectiveness in controlling some autoimmune conditions.

5. Discuss your condition with a stem cell doctor who has experience in treating your particular condition. Ask which stem cells will be used and how they will be applied to benefit your individual condition.

CHAPTER 11

Stem Cells in Autism, Stroke, MS, and Alzheimer's Disease

The future is in the mind.

Are We There Yet?

Relatively common neurological conditions seen today are autism in kids, MS in middle-age people, and Alzheimer's and other forms of dementia in the elderly. Age groups can overlap. Other disabling conditions like epilepsy and stroke can happen at any age. Neurological conditions take a toll, on not only the patients but also their immediate family.

Unfortunately, we do not know the cause of the most severe conditions. No cures are available. Most of the current treatments focus on symptom control only. The most challenging problem is that brain cells do not easily regenerate. Any brain damage or injury usually leads to permanent scarring. Stem cell therapy seems to have the potential to develop new brain cells. They also seem to be able to regenerate the cells that have been affected by the damage. However, this cannot be taken lightly.

Stem cell therapy for the brain is not as simple as the same therapy for your painful knees. For neurological conditions, we need cells that are going to help regenerate the brain. There are several clinical trials and research studies around the world currently focused on treating these conditions. The brain has many different types of cells. In each condition, the affected cell type may vary. For neurological conditions, stem cells are needed that can stimulate the nervous system to grow and replace the particular damaged brain cells. In order to produce successful results, more laboratory testing and programming of the stem cells may be required. Whether from your own body or from an external source (embryonic, umbilical cord), the stem cells will have to be programmed. This will allow them to regenerate or replace damaged brain cells.

A lot of commercial clinics claim cures for these conditions. Unfortunately, they use the same stem cells as are used in the therapies for painful joints. This is wrong. Patients get tempted by the promise of a cure and are willing to spend a lot of money. If you or your loved one is seeking stem cell treatment for a neurological condition, talk to the experts. Seek a clinical trial at a university medical center. Ask the people at the center to explain the treatment process. Try to understand what kind of stem cells will be used and how they will be delivered inside the brain. Let's look at the status of stem cell therapy in a few of these conditions.

Stem Cells and Autism

Autism is a spectrum of disorders in which affected individuals lack social and communication skills. These symptoms are coupled with repetitive behaviors and interests in only a few activities. The degree to which each of these is affected varies among different individuals on the spectrum. Current treatments include behavioral, occupational, and speech therapies. For excessive behaviors, a wide variety of psychiatric medications may be used. There is no cure today.

CASE STUDY: **BRIAN**

Brian is an 18-year-old who was diagnosed with autism at the age of 3. He seemed to be doing well physically, but his parents became concerned when he was unable to keep up with his developmental milestones. The diagnosis shocked Brian's parents, who had previously never heard of autism. They had no idea the impact it was going to have on their lives.

Brian was referred to an early intervention program. He started receiving occupational and speech therapy. Brian was a handsome kid. His appearance presented no clue to his diagnosis. He would often stare at his fingers, make little eye contact, and avoid speaking. As Brian grew into his teen years, his behavior intensified and broadened, especially into self-destructive behaviors. These involved head banging and biting. Over 15 years, Brian's parents tried all available therapies including dietary modifications, IV therapy, and chelation. They even tried intensive applied behavior analysis to help him with speech and communication. They spent everything they had taking care of Brian. It is said that when you have a child with autism, it is like paying for college from day one. As Brian's behavior intensified, he was often restrained at school.

As noted above, this complex disorder has no cure. Brian is likely to live in the shadows of caregivers for the rest of his life.

It is conditions like these that make people desperate for answers. Stem cell research is at the beginning stages for kids with autism. Studies have shown a link between inflammation of brain cells and autism. There is also a link between autoimmune disorders and autism. In auto-immune disorders, the brain is attacked by the sufferer's own cells. Stem cells by nature are anti-inflammatory and also have the ability to calm your immune system. Both these actions can be helpful in children with autism. What the source of stem cells could be and their doses are yet to be determined. And how the cells will be delivered is another question. We wish the solution were easy. This is a disorder known firsthand by one of the coauthors of this book, Dr. Gaurav Goswami, physician and author, whose twin daughters have autism.

One study has reported some benefits to use the children's own stored umbilical cord cells. Initial results are encouraging, and further investigations are under way.

What about adults with autism? We have no answers yet. Stem cells hold promise, but more research is required. It is easy for parents to fall prey to some advertised stem cell treatments. The safety and efficacy of these treatments are not yet known. Autism affects every member of the autistic person's family. Follow the advice of your autism specialist and build a strong network of resources. These are all essential. Focus on providing as much support as possible. The hope is that we may start to see more stem cell–based treatments for patients with autism.

Stem Cells and Stroke

A stroke is similar to a heart attack. A blockage in blood flow to the brain leads to cell damage. A stroke is also called a "brain attack."

CASE STUDY: **ROBERT**

Robert is a 44-year-old architect. One day, while working on one of his drawings, he couldn't feel his hand. He tried to call for help but was unable to speak. He fell in his chair, and the world went blank. His secretary, Tina, walked into his office to remind him of the next meeting. She saw his body slumped in his chair. Her first thought was that he had fallen asleep. She drew close and realized something was wrong. Robert's body was leaning to one side. Saliva was dripping down the corner of his mouth. She immediately called 911 and alerted others in the office. EMS arrived. Robert was diagnosed with what seemed like a stroke.

Robert was taken to the closest medical trauma center. He could open his eyes when he arrived but experienced a severe headache. An MRI confirmed that Robert had indeed suffered a massive stroke on one side of his brain.

After a few months, Robert was working hard on his rehab. He was still unable to move his arm. Tears rolled down his cheeks when he was unable to hold his three-year-old son. But his difficulty in speaking clearly frustrated him the most. Robert was now confined to a wheelchair. Doctors said there was no guarantee of whether he would walk or use his arm ever again.

After a long convalescence, some function was recovered. Yet, after two years, Robert still wasn't the same. A friend brought him an article about stem cells and their role in the regeneration of damaged brain cells. Although the article did not specifically discuss all the details, it did pique Robert's interest. If there was a way to regenerate and repair some of his damaged brain cells, he could regain more function. Robert's own stem cells were collected. After they were processed, they were delivered in the area of damage. Robert underwent two more rounds of similar stem cell treatments over the next 14 months. Eight weeks after his first treatment, Robert started regaining strength in his legs and arms.

Today Robert walks without any assistance. One of the first things Robert did upon regaining his arm strength was to give a tight hug to his son. He could not let go.

Stem cells used for strokes are still experimental. The questions remain as with other conditions. What particular cells should be used, and how will they be delivered. Brain cells do not easily regenerate like bone and cartilage. The process required is very different. Direct implantation of stem cells into the damaged area of the brain is a complicated procedure. Exact mapping of the damaged area in your brain has to be performed before stem cells can be delivered. Whether these are embryonic, your own, or artificially grown stem cells, all need the capability of growing into brain cells. Some exciting research is also taking place in delivering stem cells in response to an acute stroke. Doctors now give clot-busting medication to minimize damage to the brain cells. In the future, your own stem cells may be delivered to the site of a stroke to help minimize damage or even start the repair and regeneration process before damage sets in.

Stem Cells and MS

Multiple sclerosis is an autoimmune condition where your own body destroys the lining of the cells in your brain and spinal cord. Women are affected twice as often as men. The disease has both active and quiet stages. There is also continued progressive damage to neuron cells. It worsens with time. Currently, there is no cure.

CASE STUDY: **KYLE**

Kyle is a 43-year-old practicing dermatologist. He started notic-ing that he had blurry vision along with a loss of sharpness and contrast. Even after rest, his eyes would hurt. Some days were better than others. But his vision was becoming a more frequent problem. Kyle underwent a complete ophthalmological exam. His eye doctor friend was smart enough to recommend an MRI. Kyle had inflammation in his optic nerves (the nerves that control the eyes and are located behind the eyeballs), a symptom of multiple sclerosis. Kyle also had active spots of MS in both his brain and spinal cord.

In MS, as the lining of the nerves is destroyed, the conduction of the signal along the network of brain cells becomes erratic. This leads to a host of symptoms. Among them are vision loss, pain, fatigue, and impaired coordination. The symptom severity and duration can vary from person to person. Some people may be symptom-free for most of their lives, while others can have severe chronic problems that never go away.

Most treatments are based on physical therapy and immune suppression. These weaken the patient further, destroy the body, and can be extremely toxic. Current research focuses on the regeneration and repair of the nerve tract lining.

Stem cells have the potential of controlling the immune sys-tem as well as reducing inflammation. These changes can help the nerves heal. Stem cells have been used experimentally in MS patients. The cells have been derived from the patient's own bone marrow and fat as well as from embryonic and artificially enhanced stem cells, Before new stem cells are given, the old bad cells that have been attacking brain cells have to be destroyed.

This process itself can be toxic, but preliminary results are encouraging. Stem cells are showing immense promise in patients with MS and should be explored as an option.

Stem Cells and Alzheimer's

Dementia as a group of disorders is characterized by a progressive decline in brain function. Memory loss is considered a common symptom. But there are other areas of brain function that are also affected. These include critical thinking and analysis. As well, there are functions that include disconnection from emotions, and these are equally affected.

There are different forms of dementia. Alzheimer's is obviously the most common. The cause is unknown, but age, genetics, and environmental factors may be responsible. The extent to which every patient is affected depends on the type of dementia and that individual's health.

The impact Alzheimer's can have on the autonomy of the patient and his or her family members is tremendous. To watch a loved one, near and dear, slowly disappear is devastating. Family members are heartbroken when they gradually lose someone they have known and loved for so many years. This is one of the most discouraging parts of Alzheimer's disease.

Alzheimer's is often considered a condition affecting the elderly. Research now shows symptoms can start as early as the third or fourth decade of life. During old age, the loss of memory and a decrease in functional capacity are pretty remarkable. Alzheimer's is more than just memory loss.

Alzheimer's causes a decline in overall functional cognitive ability. Along with memory loss, the patient loses the ability to formulate meaningful actions, let alone execute them. Alzheimer's can cause profound changes in a person's mood and behavior. A person with Alzheimer's can become depressed, delusional, and angry for no reason. More information and resources are now available to help combat Alzheimer's. It is important to have an extremely strong network of people around you. It is also very important for the family to talk about what is happening and network with those in similar situations. Connecting with your local Alzheimer's Association chapter can be a good starting point.

Additionally, it is important to understand how Alzheimer's sufferers change over time. They won't be the same person you once knew. This can be a very hard adjustment. Educating the community is equally important. People with Alzheimer's and other forms of dementia are vulnerable to abuse and neglect. In the beginning stages of the disease, they are often misunderstood. Long before Alzheimer's patients are institutionalized or are under 24/7 care, they can seem very odd to others. The uninformed may even mistreat them. One Alzheimer's sufferer was arrested at a supermarket because he walked away without paying. A woman walked naked at night and was labeled a witch. These patients get arrested or even beaten up because of the misunderstanding of the disease.

No Cure for Alzheimer's Yet

There is no stem cell treatment for Alzheimer's presently. Researchers are working with a variety of stem cells to see which ones would be best to regenerate and repair the brain. Also, several areas of the brain and different types of brain cells may be affected in Alzheimer's. Finding stem cells that can develop into different brain cells in Alzheimer's is a major challenge. How these cells can then be delivered into various areas of the brain, as mentioned before, is another significant hurdle that needs to be overcome. Some research is focused on developing proteins lost in the brain cells of Alzheimer's patients. Finding any relief for these patients will be a major step forward. In the meantime, stay focused on proper caregiver support and maintain the good general health of any Alzheimer's family member you might have.

Light at the End

No cure yet exists for autism, stroke, MS, Alzheimer's, other dementias, or Parkinson's disease. These neurological conditions take a heavy toll not only on the patients but also on their caregivers. Significant amounts of resources, time, money, and emotions are invested in taking care of these patients. These conditions can get extremely frustrating unless one has a proper support system. Although much awareness has developed in the field of neurological conditions in the last two decades, still more needs to be accomplished. Even as we look for a cure, we should continue to provide better treatments. Most therapies are going to be in the form of occupational social speech and behavior interventions.

One good reason for hope is that the majority of these conditions involve an inflammatory process in the brain cells and immune imbalance in the immune system. Stem cells are known both to be a natural anti-inflammatory and to be capable of balancing the immune environment. This gives us tremendous hope that we will one day have successful stem cell treatments for neurological conditions. In the meantime, beware of stem cell treatments offered by some commercial providers. These will not help your loved ones. You should not spend time and money on these bogus treatments. Today you're much better off spending resources on better care and support for your loved ones. Stem cell treatments for these types of conditions are going to be technically complicated and challenging. They are not as easy as stem cell injections for joint pain.

KEY TAKEAWAYS

1. Stem cell research for autism, stroke, MS, and Alzheimer's disease is at the beginning stages.

2. What kind of stem cells? How many? How will they be delivered? These questions have not been answered yet when it comes to neurological conditions.

3. If you are interested in stem cell treatment for these conditions, look for a university-run clinical trial.

4. Your best bet today is to focus on improving the quality of life for yourself and your loved one affected by one of the above conditions.

5. Maintain hope. There is yet no cure, but we will get there soon.

CHAPTER 12

Healing from Within

A thousand prescriptions—easy.
One single remedy—hard.

Your Unique Body, Your Unique Cells

Two patients can undergo the same procedure with entirely opposite outcomes. Why? Our physical structures may appear to be the same, but physiologically and even anatomically they are different. Even when our physiology and anatomy are optimal, the state of one's mind adds another dimension. Healing is tied to the optimal functioning of both body and mind. It is very important to keep your body at optimal health, both physically and mentally. Poor diet and lack of exercise lead to a decline in physical health. Further, the trials and tribulations in life, along with their associated stress, all diminish our body's natural healing capacity. Abnormalities set in. These translate into symptoms often addressed with drugs and surgeries. This sets up a never-ending vicious cycle of doctor visits. Often the root causes are ignored.

Many more symptoms arise as side effects of the medications we are prescribed. Unwanted surgical trauma causes more damage as our quality of life declines. What can we do to avoid falling into this trap? How can we maximize every second of our journey? What a shame it would be to fall prey to avoidable illnesses that take away the joy of life. The good news is, there are many things in our control that we can do on a daily basis. We can avoid deadly illnesses and more fully enjoy our lives.

Job #1: Take Care of Your Body

Several research studies have shown that aging is sped up by inflammation and stress. Both wear your cells and cause premature cell death. The same studies have shown that restricting caloric intake and engaging in exercise can counter or at least slow down the aging process in your cells. Even though your genetic makeup influences your health, there is also a lot you can still control.

As our understanding of stem cells improves, we will be able to focus on how best we can heal ourselves. The medical community has long talked about treating the patient as a whole. Yet several mainstream treatments—medications and surgeries—focus only on symptom relief without inducing any true healing. As patients, we seek help for symptoms. These symptoms are a manifestation of underlying problems, impacting how our cells function. These underlying problems need to be addressed. In addition to any treatment, it is important that we take care of our bodies. If our bodies are healthy, we can avoid many of these problems. Staying healthy requires a daily routine that focuses on our physical and mental well-being. For any treatment to work best, our bodies have to be otherwise healthy. We often connect with patients treated years earlier. In most cases, those who have experienced long-term relief took good care of their bodies. As much as a physician would like to take credit, the credit for real long-term healing success goes to these patients. The treatments were successful because the patients were committed to leading a healthy life.

Our bodies are the most complex machines ever developed. If you want any piece of equipment to perform properly, you need to maintain it well. You take great care of your car ensuring that it performs its best. You don't want any unexpected breakdowns.

Similarly, your body works in unison with many other parts and systems. Your heart beats continually until your last moment. All systems are in constant need of the right kind of nourishment to perform optimally. This nourishment comes in the form of your environment, thoughts, and obviously what you eat. They are all equally important.

Other Factors

Healing also depends upon your genetics, the nature of the injury, the location of the injury, and the particular organ involved. We can debate the various causes and factors that lead to disease and injury. What predisposes us to disease or even injury is still largely unknown, and the answer probably lies in our genes. Two individuals living in the same environment with similar lifestyles can develop very different diseases. The difference in why someone is more likely to suffer from a particular condition is still beyond our understanding and control. Similarly, how well we respond to treatments (including stem cells) is also determined in part by our genes.

As noted above, the site of injury or disease is also a factor. Tissues do not all carry the same regenerative capacity. Different organs and their cells have different inherent capacities to regenerate, replicate, and differentiate. This can impact healing. These are factors beyond our control. Different methods of treatment, different types of stem cells, and varying interventions might be needed to address a particular organ or individual. Treatments have to be and should be customized.

Because these factors are beyond your control, it is extremely important that you stay focused on controlling your general health and well-being. For example, inflammation throughout the body is rampant in obesity. Even the best of treatments may not get optimal results. Lack of proper cell function not only delays healing but will likely lead to further disease and misery. What can you do?

Regeneration, Repair, and Healing

There are certain things that can help your body stay in an optimal state. Obviously, if you suffer from certain deficiencies or medical disorders, you have to follow your mainstream doctor's advice. In addition, there are other things you can do on a daily basis that can help keep your body in peak state. These daily recommendations also help your cells stay healthy. When your cells are healthy and energized, your body will optimize its healing power. Nothing works in a week or two. For long-term results, you have to develop daily healthy habits. Your car comes with a maintenance plan; your body has one too.

There are six simple recommendations backed by years of research. These six items are known to play a role in regeneration, repair, and healing. They might appear to be simple, but if you can commit yourself to these six steps daily, your body is going to need very little outside help. Let's list them here, and we will review each in greater detail as we move forward.

1. Maintain hydration.
2. Cut down on sugar intake.
3. Eat pomegranates.
4. Eat walnuts.
5. Provide daily heat therapy to the body parts that hurt.
6. Move, exercise, do yoga, do deep breathing, or meditate.

The great six (or as we like to say, G6) promote healing and regeneration. But as mentioned above, the G6 is recommended not only for when you are injured or need a procedure. These recommendations are fundamental enough to form habits and daily rituals. If you do these every day, cells (including your stem cells) will be in an optimal state ready for regeneration and repair anytime your body is attacked by disease or injury. Merely wanting a healthy body or a calm mind will not work by itself. Nothing happens unless you do positive things. But once you take action, your body will become its own pharmacy. Your body will heal itself naturally. It will become your own temple, your own retreat of joy and happiness. Now that is what we call "true healing."

CASE STUDY: **RAYMOND**

Raymond is a 94-year-old who has danced all his life. For the past four years, he has started to slow down. This was due to constant pain in his right hip. Raymond visited several doctors and was not considered a surgical candidate given his age. He was offered pain medication and cortisone injections. In addition, he was told to forget about ever dancing again. Raymond wanted to die on the dance floor—that's how much he loved dancing. But none of the treatments guaranteed he could continue.

Raymond was otherwise very healthy. He maintained normal body weight, and he had no heart disease or diabetes. His friend

had a shoulder problem years earlier treated with stem cell therapy. He advised Raymond to go see the same doctor in hopes of
finding some relief. Raymond had advanced wear-and-tear damage
to his right hip joint. He was treated with an injection of his own
stem cells. A month later, Raymond started to go for long walks
and engaged in physical therapy. Four months after treatment, he
was back dancing at his social club. He became a crowd favorite
once again, with his moves still pleasing the ladies.

One would think at 94 there would be little chance of regeneration and repair. A healthy body plus a healthy mind promotes
stem cell regeneration. This also produces a chance for longer
life. Raymond's stem cells were strong enough for the process of
regeneration and repair. He had a good outcome because he had
taken good care of his body.

Habits for Health

Let's explore our G6 recommendations in more detail.

Hydration

Your body is 70% water. Coincidentally, the planet is also 70%
water. Hydration is essential to cellular functions. Many studies
have shown the benefits of hydration. Most impactful has been
research on patients with lower back problems. Low back pain sufferers were divided into two groups. Group 1 was given hydration.
The people in this group were ordered to drink up to one gallon of
water throughout the day. Group 2 had no such intervention. They
were only told to continue their basic lifestyle. After six weeks, low

back pain scores dropped in the well-hydrated group by 50%. This was huge.

Low back pain can be very tricky to manage. No surgery or therapy can guarantee a 50% reduction in back pain. As the cells that make up your spine become hydrated, the regenerative process speeds up. Healthy and well-hydrated disks provide the cushion necessary to support the spine. This is just one profound example of what hydration can do for your body. Hydration helps cells function well. A well-hydrated body gets rid of toxins more easily. Our environment, food, and inflammatory processes due to injury and disease all build toxins. These toxins cause us pain and other symptoms. Hydration is an easy way of flushing these toxins out of your body.

Another benefit of hydration is its impact on your blood and circulation. When you are dehydrated, your blood becomes too dense and thick. Blood that is thicker tends to move slowly through your blood vessels.

This slow flow increases the risk that certain abnormal cells, cholesterol, and fat will stick to the vessel walls.

This is even more likely to happen when the vessel walls themselves are inflamed. The risk of vessel wall blockage increases. All of this causes poor circulation and further spreads inflammation throughout your body. All the more reason to stay well hydrated!

Sugar Intake

You have probably had experience with both low-fat and nonfat diets. Your dieting likely has had little impact on your health. We have become more obese as a nation! The real answer to weight loss is decreasing sugar intake. Excess sugar circulating in the body gets converted to fat. This leads to weight gain. Sugar induces the release of insulin. This hormone can create a lot of inflammation. As you know, inflammation causes the whole body to become more painful. When undergoing a procedure, patients with diabetes or high blood sugar tend to experience a lot more pain and discomfort compared with patients with normal sugar levels. This is due to a generalized state of inflammation in their bodies.

Sugar is an immediate body fuel that is useful when exercising at the gym. Sugar is a necessary fuel when playing any sports. Sugar gets burned off with exercise and intense physical activity. But the majority of us tend not to spend much time engaging in physical activity. Most of us are occupied with work and have a sedentary lifestyle. This leads to sugar accumulating in the body, forming fat and causing inflammation. This also creates a vicious cycle. The more unused sugar, the more the body packs it into fat. Think of sugar as a checking account and fat as savings. When you move extra money from your checking account to your savings account, your body converts unused sugar into fat. Perhaps a fatter dollar savings account is a good thing. But more fat in your body never is. To reverse this cycle, fat needs to be broken down. You want to deprive your body of external sugar. Your body will break down fat to provide sugar when needed. That can happen only when you stop consuming extra sugar. There are plenty of weight-loss fads and gimmicks. But pure weight loss only comes from decreasing sugar intake and maintaining the fat-burning process. This "sugar conversion into fat" concept is very important in understanding how your body works.

Pomegranates

Pomegranate supplements can be beneficial. They can assist your body in regeneration and repair. Unfortunately, by the time any nutrient is packed in a bottle, it has already started to lose efficacy. A lot of what we buy, even when labeled as 100% natural, is not. Nature has an abundance of helpful nutritious products. Two of these, based on significant research, are pomegranate fruit and walnuts. The pomegranate is a tropical fruit rich in antioxidants. As noted in an earlier chapter, it also helps provide nitric oxide buildup. Nitric oxide, not to be confused with nitrous oxide used in dental anesthesia, is a chemical that helps relax blood vessels and improves blood flow. Studies have shown how pomegranate juice provides cells with substantial amounts of nitric oxide to help treat many disorders.

Pomegranates are not the only natural source of nitric oxide. Another source is beets. But a downside of beets can be an elevation of blood sugar. Pomegranate juice actually helps lower blood sugar. In one study of diabetic patients eating pomegranates, hemoglobin A1C (a marker of average blood sugar level) was lowered.

Pomegranates also help patients with diabetes gain better control of their disease. The benefits of pomegranates translate into an improved circulation throughout your body. It lowers bad cholesterol and blood pressure. As we age, nitric oxide production in our body drops. It is extremely important we rebuild it using pomegranates. Nitric oxide helps relax our blood vessels thereby improving blood flow.

Walnuts

Walnuts are a tremendous source of omega-3s. Walnuts also have a beneficial effect on promoting nitric oxide formation, discussed above. Omega-3 fatty acids help stabilize cell membranes throughout the body. They help reduce inflammation in the lining of our joints. Omega-3 is also found in seafood. Unfortunately, ocean-caught seafood is becoming contaminated. These sources can no longer be trusted to be healthy. In fact, few supplements containing omega-3 can be trusted due to varying levels of contaminants found in commercial products. Trust natural sources instead. It is much safer to grab a handful of walnuts. And while to some, they are not the greatest tasting by themselves, they can be added to any food throughout the day. A lot of patients sprinkle the nuts on their meals.

Heat

Heat versus cold is the eternal debate! Both feel good at the skin level. Cold ice packs are common among athletes to reduce swelling and inflammation. They also are a way to restrict blood flow to an injured area. Ice works short term. It shuts down blood flow. It is recommended immediately after injury or surgery to minimize bleeding. If there is bleeding at the site of a fresh injury, the inflammatory response can be more pronounced. However, after 24 to 48 hours after an acute injury, heat therapy is better because it causes the blood vessels to relax and improve the blood flow to the area. Improved blood flow brings in more nutrition and washes out the toxins released by damaged cells.

Generally speaking, heat therapy is good once the acute phase is over. With heat you are trying to provide more blood flow, leading to more healing. Some experts recommend alternating heat and cold; again a lot of this comes down to a personal choice for some people. Scientifically, heat therapy is better at promoting regeneration and repair as well as alleviating chronic pain.

Several patients have been able to manage their pain better and wean themselves off dangerous pain medications by creating a heating routine. As little as 20 minutes applying a heating pad to the affected area can do wonders to decrease pain. You can also use an old-fashioned hot-water bottle or a rice heating pad, warmed up in the microwave. The problem is that such methods do not deliver consistent heat. It's worth investing in a good $20 heating pad available from your local pharmacy. Many come with a timer and intensity adjustments. A heating pad provides the injured and painful area with consistent heat. You can repeat this process as many times as you want. There is a caution before applying a heating pad. Make sure your skin is clean and dry. Make sure you remove topical ointments or other local pain applications. Wipe the skin dry before applying the heating pad. The combination of heat and local skin applications can lead to skin irritation and even cause burns.

One of the authors (also a patient) of this book, Kerry Johnson, experienced pain at the thoracic 11 level of the midback for years. To quote him, "Before stem cell therapy, the only relief was ice. Icing my back was a consistent habitual activity after every tennis match. In fact, 50% of my tennis club buddies ice some part of their body immediately after leaving the court." But pain often returned within a few hours. Few tennis players know the benefits of heat. Many can't play more than a couple of times a week. If they had a regular heat regimen, match play could be a lot more frequent and comfortable. Heat relaxes the local muscles and improves blood flow to the area. Heat also washes away local toxins, thus promoting repair. Heat makes a huge difference when pain is more severe and chronic. Heat can help once the initial risk of bleeding is gone.

Move–Exercise–Slow and Deep Breathing–Meditate

Move and exercise daily. Breathe deeply in a quiet area. Power-walk. Go to the gym. All have been shown to be beneficial. But you have to make a commitment. Taking slow deep breaths has significant benefits and serves as the first step in any yoga. Deep breathing maximizes the oxygen supply to your body. It is also important to support your body's physical structure, especially the alignment of the spine. Focusing on one's breathing is one of the easiest ways to meditate.

It truly does not matter what type of exercise you do as long as you feel the positive flow of energy. Find any physical activity that you like and just do it. The most important thing is having a daily routine. When it comes to any form of physical activity or exercise routine you adopt, remember consistency is more important than intensity. It should take no more than 20 to 30 minutes. But do it daily.

A gym owner once told me only 33% of paying members exercise regularly. In fact, when gyms are built, this low attendance is factored into their size. They sell more memberships than the gym can handle. The only time the facility is crowded is in January and early February. This is appalling. There are people willing to pay without using what they signed up for. Let's reverse that trend.

Commit to keeping your body moving. Any activity or exercise will be helpful. Mix and match your exercises. Get creative with your routines. Pay attention to your muscles. Work on a different body area on different days. Muscle confusion (avoiding the same exercises every day) is a proven path to fitness. Give your muscles enough time to rest and recover. Unless you are working toward a specific goal, keep an evenly balanced workout.

Stretching is important. A really good idea is to stretch when you wake up and before you go to bed. Muscles lose 30% of their mass as you age. With muscle loss comes joint discomfort. Minor joint pain is often relieved with a simple but consistent stretch.

A pro golfer once told me that every player on tour does something no amateurs even think of. The players stretch. Even the famous Arnold Palmer would stretch before hitting on a driving range. He would hold his chipping wedge horizontally while turning his torso to each side as far as the stretch would take him. A good stretch is with resistance. You can use a rubber strap on the edge of your bed to provide some tension. This resistance will help stretch as well as tone. Stretching will also prevent common injuries.

If you play a sport, make sure you cross-train in other sports. This can help more muscles stay conditioned in case you make an awkward motion while playing your chosen sport. You can suffer if your body is not physically conditioned.

The Body Follows the Mind

No amount of healthy nutrition, environment, exercise, or medical procedures can make you healthy. Not even stem cell therapies can work unless your mind is focused. Your mind controls the body. Your perception of the world and how you react to it are critical in maintaining optimal physical health. In our experience after looking at outcomes of thousands of procedures, we determined that the best results are experienced by patients who have a mindset of maintaining their physical and mental health. These are also patients who have learned to lower their stress and stay positive. Several studies show the physical health-stress connection.

Those with an active exercise regimen including any form of mental health release have lower levels of stress. Mental maintenance can be playing a game of chess, reading a good book, or even taking a walk with your family. In fact, that last activity can help both your mental and physical health. Most of us fail to maintain our physical and mental health. This maintenance is often difficult because of constant distraction. In this world of

24/7 news and social media, your mind can be an advocate or an enemy of health. Controlling your mind comes from focus. You are going to have distractions. But you need to stay focused on what's important and lock in like a missile on your health goals.

Create a Body That Heals Itself

Your main goal and focus in life should be to stay healthy. That should be the overriding thought taking precedence over everything you do. Your health is the big picture. Pay attention to your health first. You cannot enjoy what life has to offer unless you are healthy. When you first try to change habits, you may fail—we all fail. Many patients struggle in the beginning to develop healthy habits. It's like learning to ride a bicycle. Only by repeated attempts can you stay on the bike. Stay focused on your healthy habits. Your health is the prize. True happiness is an alignment between your thoughts and actions. The more you can ignore the distractions, the happier you will be. The more you focus on your health and stay disciplined, the easier it will become. Push through the distractions and short-term discomfort. Your physical health and mental health are interrelated. Work on both every day. Use these pointers to manage your mind and body better.

We end this section with a cautionary tale. Have you heard about the yoga instructor who suffered a stroke while performing a difficult handstand for her students? A few years earlier, a model suffered a stroke following a neck manipulation by her chiropractor. Both women were young. Both suffered a tear in an artery supplying blood to their brain. One was lucky to survive. The model lost her life. Both cases highlight how delicate our bodies are. One should not push the limits. No exercise is worth an injury. At the same time, even though the yoga teacher's stroke was a pretty scary event, she made a full recovery. She credited it to her body's ability to heal quickly. Her daily practice of yoga and healthy eating also helped. So did meditation, which has been a vital part of her yoga routine. Meditation helped her get through the ordeal. It helped her mentally stay strong. Her healthy habits helped her recover faster.

Studies have shown that patients with normal body weight and without other medical conditions recover much faster after an injury or surgery. In comparison, patients with compromised health recover poorly following a similar injury or surgery. These patients have a longer recovery period. Their outcomes are also worsened.

Assistive Technologies

You may have experienced or heard about light therapy (photo-biomodulation), laser therapy, cryotherapy, electromagnetic therapy, adaptive conditioning, etc. There is no conclusive evidence of the effectiveness of these treatments for any particular condition. Most of these technologies have been around for years and are generally considered safe. Several athletes use them to gain any competitive advantage they may offer. Some are purely used as rest and recovery tools. Photo-biomodulation involving different intensities of red, blue, and infrared light therapy is probably the most studied. Patients have reported benefits when it's applied correctly using the right device. It's known to activate the mitochondria (the energy powerhouse in our cells), thereby helping repair and regeneration.

Most of the time applications of these devices suffer due to lack of standardized methods. Even though the underlying technology is proven, the devices created may not be effectively applying science and technology. Newer products are always being introduced in the field of sports medicine. You should evaluate the science behind these devices and products. Always ask what role the product would play in your condition. Is there potential for harm? Do not buy into the hype and expect miracles, only to be disappointed later.

KEY TAKEAWAYS

We all have a list of what is important to us. Here again are our G6 (G for "great") scientific recommendations that will help keep your stem cells healthy and happy, thereby helping you lead a productive life:

1. Maintain hydration.
2. Cut down on your sugar intake.
3. Eat pomegranates.
4. Eat walnuts.
5. Apply daily heat therapy to injured body parts.
6. Move, exercise, breathe deeply, meditate.

How many of the above G6 are you doing daily?

CHAPTER 13

Stem Cells and the FDA

Steroids, pharmaceutical drugs, and surgery are legal,
but they can hurt a lot of people.

The Coming Stem Cell Regulation

Just as all politics is local, all regulation is local. Several countries in Europe, South America, and Asia have taken the lead with certain stem cell treatments. Part of the problem with stem cell technologies is the numerous types of stem cells. Also, a host of sources are available for stem cells, both foreign and your own. Further, the methods of isolating the cells are extremely variable. How they are processed and delivered may also vary. This has made the regulatory process unpredictable. The treatment itself is subject to various interpretations.

Any new treatment is expected to be met with a certain degree of skepticism. Stem cells are likely to face even more resistance from organized medicine. One of the main reasons is because stem cell treatments are not pharmaceutically driven, at least not yet. Traditionally a pharmaceutical company or device manufacturer will first get its product approved by the FDA. The next step is getting insurance coverage approval. Once these approvals are in place, the industry will then approach doctors and other providers, offering training on that product. All these steps have nothing to do with the efficacy of the product!

The FDA has served as a benchmark for a lot of other countries, though it has had its own challenges. In 2018, the FDA issued recalls, withdrawals from the market, or safety alerts for more than 300 products.

CASE STUDY: **KRISTIN**

Kristin, an active social media consultant, was diagnosed with rheumatoid arthritis when she was 38 years old. She was frightened when she found out there was no cure. She would have to live with the disease. Rheumatoid arthritis (RA) affects 1% of the world's population and is different from the more common wear-and-tear osteoarthritis that the majority suffer from. It is more commonly seen in women. RA is an autoimmune condition. Your own body reacts to the lining of the joints, causing inflammation, pain, and deformity. The World Health Organization (WHO) estimates that within 10 years of its onset, half of the patients are unable to hold a full-time job. Being young and at the height of her successful career, Kristin was determined to do everything in her power to keep her RA under control.

Her first goal was to keep her pain and inflammation in her joints in check. At about the same time, her doctor mentioned the availability of a new drug without the side effects of traditionally used arthritic medications. Kristin was aware that commonly used painkillers and other RA medications can cause heart attacks, heart failure, and stroke. In fact, just a few years before her diagnosis, there was a major recall of a commonly prescribed painkiller. The medication was withdrawn because it caused sudden deaths. Kristin's doctor said the new drug had been recently approved by the FDA and was being hailed for its excellent safety profile. Kristin started receiving (IV) injection treatments of this medication every month.

In the third month, following two doses of the injection, Kristin noticed some odd symptoms she had never experienced before. She had bouts of palpitations as her heart raced and trembling of her hands due to tremors. She also occasionally experienced shortness of breath. When she reported the symptoms to her doctor, she was told it was not related to the medication. Over the next two months, Kristin continued to feel the symptoms. She was told they were possibly related to anxiety. The doctor recommended that she seek psychotherapy. Around the same time, another patient receiving the same medication reported the same symptoms on a social media post. Her doctor told her the same thing—that these were not the side effects of this medication. None of these symptoms were listed on the drug label.

Soon a report emerged of a 70-year-old man suffering a fatal brain bleed two days after receiving an IV injection of this medication. This was followed by another report of a woman in her 60s suffering a heart attack after starting the same medication. It soon became clear that a significant number of people were reporting side effects.

A medication that claimed not to have the side effects compared with its competitor drugs probably caused the same side effects. It wasn't safer than its competitors. Both the patients and their providers were misled. Regulation in this case failed. The reason was that long-term studies require years of data to be collected. Rarely does the FDA have that information before approval is granted. In the meantime, there is little to prevent pharmaceutical companies from making false claims.

Applications of stem cells shift the framework of how medicine is practiced and has been for decades. There is no involvement of pharmaceutical or device companies when dealing with your own cells. In fact, the goal of stem cell treatments is to keep you away from drugs. This eliminates some very powerful middlemen. A further complication is the third-party healthcare system. The system makes it more challenging for patients to try out treatments not backed by powerful pharmaceutical companies. It is likely that in the coming years, we may see even more restrictions on the application of your own stem cells, especially in the United States.

Medical Tourism

Today it is easier to travel the world. But social media and the internet have made the world one common playground. Ideas, thoughts, and stories get quickly exchanged. The same thing happens in the world of stem cells. Somebody goes to a treatment center. The person experiences a fabulous result, and then people blindly line up at that center. No one knows if it was fake or real news. Even if one particular treatment was effective, it would not be for every medical condition or even for each patient. That is not how it works when it comes to stem cells. So, beware of what you learn on the internet.

One of the biggest problems is when local regulators fail to act in your own country. It then promotes medical tourism. Patients are desperate to seek solutions, especially when mainstream medicine has failed. They will seek and are promised treatments that have no scientific basis. The regulatory framework in other countries may be weak or have very little oversight. It is extremely important that regulators work to standardize the collection and application of stem cells. Millions of consumers are at risk of being scammed by for-profit clinics in foreign countries with little or no legal recourse. Your best bet is to understand the treatment you are being promised. Seek multiple opinions from other stem cell providers as well as run everything by your own primary doctor. Your own doctor knows you best.

Areas of Concern

With anything new, regulations tend to lag. Without regulation, practices develop without proper oversight. The major question facing all of us in the world of stem cells (which the FDA will consider) is the manipulation of cells in their biological form. Biological manipulation is how stem cells are isolated from harvested tissue, regardless of the source. The next question is, Are the stem cells then stimulated to multiply or grow into a certain type of tissue? These methods and processes are the ones that need to be understood in great detail. One needs to fully understand these procedures and the impact they will have on the cell function. Could there be a potential for introducing harm once the manipulated cells are implanted in your body? This is the single most important area of debate right now among the regulators.

You may have heard about the Chinese investigator who manipulated a gene sequence by deleting a gene in the embryonic stage in order to protect a baby from certain infections. However, deleting a gene could also have other unintended consequences. When we treat a patient with medications, surgery, or the patient's own stem cells, both good and bad effects are limited to that individual. When we start altering the genetic makeup of a cell, the impact could be felt for generations to come. The same thing applies to cloning. One has to be extremely careful in dealing with cells and biological tissue. We have no idea of the potential consequences.

This creates a dilemma, especially among the general public. All stem cell treatments carry the same title. What is the impact that laboratory manipulation can have on stem cells? Also, as clinical applications advance, the question will be how to optimize the role of stem cells for a specific condition. Clearly, for certain complex conditions, stem cells will have to be programmed to perform certain functions and grow into a particular cell type. It is naive to assume stem cells that work to grow your cartilage and meniscus will also work to grow your brain cells! All of this raises important questions for regulators. A lot of due diligence is required. Answers may not be easy to come by. Besides regulators, providers also bear responsibility. Physicians offering stem cell treatments should be clear about their methods and processes. All parties need to help formulate guidelines for standardization and implementation. Unfortunately, that rarely happens. Currently, regulators, scientists, and practicing physicians are at great odds when it comes to stem cell treatments. Sometimes, however, the only problem may be that they are not speaking the same language.

Unlike with medications, we haven't reached a stage with stem cells where we can really figure out how many cells are needed to treat a particular condition. Knowing stem cell counts may be important. And more important is knowing how many of those cells are alive. You are dealing with live biological tissue. If, for some reason, during the collection, isolation, or processing stage the stem cells die, it doesn't matter what the count was. Effective treatment can only be determined once there are enough data on both cell count and viability.

There is an unfortunate trend among commercial suppliers of foreign cells of charging customers based on the number of cells provided. However, no one really knows how many cells you need in the first place. Even if you purchase a high number of cells, what really matters is how many of those cells are really alive. As you can see, regulators have their work cut out for them. Every aspect of stem cell treatment needs to be parsed.

Recently there was a spate of infections in patients treated with umbilical cord tissue. Several patients had to be hospitalized. Foreign sources of cells are a significant area of concern. This begins with donor screening. Whom are you collecting stem cells from? How thoroughly has their medical history and background been vetted? Were any tests performed to exclude infection? How were the cells collected and transported? How were the cells processed in the laboratory? Were the cells expanded or multiplied? How were the cells readied for their ultimate use? All this needs to be thoroughly vetted. These are all serious questions that currently have no answer. This is one area where regulation should be a top priority. The so-called biopharmaceutical companies will now replace pure pharmaceutical companies. They will treat stem cells in the same manner as they do with drugs. They will submit short-term white paper studies with insufficient subjects to convince the FDA to get approval. Unfortunately, the more things change, the more they remain the same.

Understanding at the Cellular Level

For treatments to be approved, the FDA needs to focus on how it views disease and injury. We know in any disease or injury there is local cell destruction. All damage occurs at the cell level. If we are really going to treat disease and injury, we have to make local cells healthy and functional. This is what is meant by having a cellular viewpoint. It is understanding disease and injury at a cellular level.

The FDA is still looking at organ systems structurally rather than at the cellular level. For example, in the FDA's November 2017 report, questions were raised about using fat inside the joint! Fat clearly doesn't belong in joint space. Many stem cell experts would agree to that. But the justification is that fat serves as an easily collectible source of your stem cells. Fat cells are condensed oil and should be discarded. Isolated stem cells are what you need. When removed correctly, fat lends itself to providing a large source of stem cells without compromising your body. People have never complained that a physician removed too much fat from their body! The FDA described fat as a tissue that is supposed to support and provide a cushion between organ systems. Because of that role, it has no place inside a joint. This is clearly a structural viewpoint and misses the fact that your fat is merely being used as an easily dispensable source of your own stem cells.

Bone marrow, blood, muscle, and joint lining are all sources of stem cells. In fact, virtually every organ in your body contains stem cells. As discussed, fat tissue is made up of many kinds of cells. This includes millions of mesenchymal (fat) stem cells. Since these cells can be collected in large amounts, potentially millions of your own stem cells can be harvested. Doctors should develop safe methods to break down fat and filter out the patient's own stem cells. This viewpoint shift from the FDA's structural aspect to a cellular one would be required to formulate solid regulatory guidelines and maximize the application of stem cells to the general public. Disease, injury, or symptoms you experience are all manifestations of cellular dysfunction. Unless your cells heal, any treatment will be ineffective. This understanding is critical to developing and regulating stem cell treatments.

Your Own Cells Should Be First

The FDA can make a positive impact if it looks into autologous sources (your own cells). Once a clear distinction is made regarding your own cells versus foreign sources, the FDA could then standardize the best collection methods. Your own stem cells can be processed during the same-day procedure, or they could be sent to a laboratory for processing. Receiving your own stem cells eliminates a host of variables one sees with foreign stem cells. With a same-day, same-sitting technique, there is less risk of altering stem cells. Also, since the cells are fresh, the cell counts are high, and more importantly so is the cell viability. But sterility can be a concern. The methods used need to be clarified and standardized. Some benchmarks will need to be developed to make sure there is more uniformity among clinics. This is one area that needs to be regulated quickly.

The power of your own stem cells is simply amazing. Your stem cells work on a daily basis already repairing and healing your body from constant wear and tear. Your own stem cells can handle 90% of the conditions that afflict you. For highly complex conditions, you will need cells from other sources. But before you go there, why not fully understand and use the potential that your own stem cells can offer. Your body is a gold mine of millions of stem cells. Your skin, teeth, and every organ inside your body have stem cells. Wouldn't you want to harness that energy and use it to repair your body? When it comes to your own stem cells, all you're doing is providing help to an area in your body that needs more help. The local cells are not able to make the repair on their own. You are just collecting stem cells from a healthy area and putting them where help is needed. What can be more natural than that?

What Can You Do?

Stem cells are not just another treatment fad. They are a whole new way of practicing medicine. Regenerative medicine is being created right in front of your eyes. The lack of standardization of stem cell treatment methods is going to make it more challenging to identify the good from the bad. Treatment, provider, and outcome variations are all over the place. Regulators should work with scientists and physicians dealing with your own stem cells to better understand how a consensus can be reached. Unless that happens, you could be reading a positive report of stem cell treatment and a negative one on the same day in the same newspaper. This is further complicated by inadequate or unethical treatments. The good work of the few is offset by the greed of others.

This lack of standardization creates a lot of skepticism among potential patients who could benefit from this therapy. In the short term, the public is likely to be left very confused trying to make treatment choices. It should be the collective responsibility of us all to help further stem cell treatments. The right questions need to be asked. Get involved with your local stem cell clinics; visit them and gain knowledge. Attend stem cell meetings and seminars. If something sounds too good to be true, it probably is. Write to local elected officials, state assembly members, and congressional representatives and senators. If you've had a positive experience, write about it. If you've had a negative one, write about it. Spread awareness. We all can benefit from properly regulated stem cell treatments.

The same applies if you carry healthcare insurance. The purpose of insurance is for you to get the best care possible. If you could benefit from a PRP injection or a stem cell knee procedure, why is an insurance company forcing you to have cortisone injections or undergo surgery? Don't settle. Ask the company why it won't approve stem cell treatment for you.

Stem cells present a unique situation. Organized medicine, big pharma, and device manufacturers are all feeling threatened. When it comes to your own stem cells, no one is lobbying for you. In fact, the FDA wants to classify stem cells as a drug—meaning you can't own your stem cells. The change will have to start from the ground up. Stem cell treatments will become mainstream only as a result of the collective will of the masses. Start questioning your physicians, local officials, regulators, and insurance companies.

KEY TAKEAWAYS

One critical question you can ask regulators and elected officials is this:

Why don't I own my own stem cells?

CHAPTER 14

A Patient's Journey with Stem Cells

Kerry Johnson's Story in His Own Words

Last hope, best hope

From Pain to Pain-Free

I have been playing tennis since I was five. My mom, Joanne Johnson, would take me to the courts behind Clackamas High School near Portland, Oregon. She would feed me balls while I flailed with an old, beat-up wooden tennis racket. In fact, I was so addicted to the sport that I would hit anything I could find, preferably a tennis ball, against our garage door for hours on end. My biggest hindrance was that there were very few kids my age to play tennis with. Most of my friends played baseball and basketball. I played those sports also, but I would have to practically bribe my friends to hit a tennis ball with me.

For the next 10 years, I played the juniors, competing in as many tournaments as I could. Transferring to the University of California, San Diego, I finally got my chance to play at the collegiate level. My family wasn't wealthy. But I was able to put myself through college by teaching tennis after class. I made $25 an hour in 1974, close to $100 an hour today. That was just enough to pay tuition. I even traded tennis lessons for room and board during the semester. Those were the golden days of tennis in the '70s.

I skipped my college graduation and traveled to Monte Carlo to compete in my first pro tournament. The clay courts were slippery, and the ball bounce seemed random. But I was able to win just enough matches during 1976–1978 to keep traveling and playing. I jokingly say now that I was ranked 95 in the world until they fixed the ATP computer ranking system where I slipped to 10,035.

I had some big wins in those days. I beat the German national champion in the first round at the Open in Munich. In Düsseldorf, my doubles partner and I went deep in the tournament.

Back in the 1970s, tennis was one of the most popular sports in the world. But it wasn't all glamour. There were low points as well. After losing in Munich, my next tournament was in Linz, Austria. I lost my wallet after the tournament in Munich and was resigned to hitchhiking the three-hour ride to Austria. I got to the Autobahn and stuck my thumb out for four hours with no luck. There was a beer garden next to the freeway. I spent the night in my sleeping bag there wondering how I would get to Linz.

In the morning, I asked the bartender for a piece of cardboard and a felt pen. I wrote in big black letters "Tennis Lehrer–Linz" and walked back out to the autobahn. The first car stopped and apologized for not taking me. He was only going to the next exit. But the driver of the next car, a Volkswagen bug, said he would take me the three hours to Linz even though he lived in Germany.

Tennis Lehrer means "tennis teacher" in German. I knew just enough German, and how crazy the Germans were about tennis, to guess they would want to meet a touring pro and get free lessons. When I arrived in Linz, I was able to borrow enough money to enter the tournament. I paid my debt after winning a few rounds and continued to play throughout my European tour.

A 22-year-old doesn't appreciate the wear and tear tennis inflicts on the body. There is a constant impact on the knees, feet, hips, and everywhere else. Because of the back arch during a kick serve, the spine torques and twists. Eventually, this all catches up. Sure, we all had aches and pains on the tour. We had elbow problems, would frequently sprain ankles, and even more often would twist knees and hips. But every 22-year-old on the tennis tour thinks he is indestructible. The body degenerates and slowly provides a painful answer for every twist, back arch, and elbow strain it has endured for decades.

A Life-Changing Event

In 2009, my 55-year-old body answered for 50 years of physical indiscretion. I gave a speech to the Hawaii Tax Institute in Honolulu, Hawaii, and came back with Type A flu. On that Monday, I traveled to New York City, speaking to an insurance company, and returned with pneumonia. On the flight later to LAX, I progressed into sepsis (blood infection). When we landed, I reached for the overhead luggage bin and collapsed on the airplane paralyzed. Triple organ failure ensued, and I was likely saved by an experimental antibiotic. After three weeks in a coma and another month in ICU, I had lost 35% of my body weight.

While I survived, spending nearly eight weeks on my back in a hospital bed proved to be the start of my spinal debilitation.

Six months after the sepsis episode, I played tennis with some friends on a Thursday night. While driving home, I felt sharp pains shooting in the middle of my back. My doting wife, Merita, drew an Epsom salt bath in hopes of providing me with some relief. But it was of little help. That evening was the start of an eight-year nightmare of pain.

Eight Years of Pain

There wasn't a day during that period that I was without pain. I've read that back pain sufferers are some of those most at risk for suicide. After experiencing that level of pain, I can understand why. Physicians say that pain is rated between 1 and 10, where 1 is discomfort and 10 is so severe that you just want someone to shoot you in the head. At worst mine was an 8. At best it never moderated below 4. But I would never give up. I still played tennis in pain, often depending on opioids to last throughout the match.

There was so much pain that my tennis skill, at a one-point pro tour level at 7.0 decreased to 4.0, the rank of a C-level player. I remember playing one doubles tournament hoping that the other team would beat us quickly so I could get off the court and out of pain. Pro athletes are the most competitive people in the world. It took a lot to drain the competition out of me. Good or bad, I was unwilling to give up the sport. I knew that if I stopped playing tennis, or working out at the gym, that would be the end.

In 2011, I saw a very exclusive orthopedic surgeon who made me wait two months for an appointment. He diagnosed several problems including bone-on-bone disks at the lower lumbar area, as well as scoliosis, a curvature of the spine. But none of that explained the intense pain at 55 years old that never bothered me earlier. He immediately prescribed spinal surgery, just like all the other doctors I'd seen.

After seeing even more surgeons, the pain was finally diagnosed locally at the 11th rib in the right thoracic area. Three doctors said there was nothing anyone could do with that area of the spine. I would just have to live with it. One physician's theory was that the ligament that connects the ribs to the spine at the T11 area was loose and pulled apart when I played tennis. He theorized that the rib would actually separate from the spine during tennis and afterward caused my excruciating pain.

Another surgeon, a friend of mine at Palisades Tennis Club in Newport Beach, California, recommended excising the rib. He actually wanted to remove the rib, thinking that supermodels do it to get hourglass figures, so why couldn't it relieve my back pain?

Soon after, I read about a disk replacement surgery called ADR. American orthopedic surgeons would replace a spinal disk with a synthetic one, providing a cushion for the spine. But since I had three damaged disks, no American doctor would do the surgery. One German doctor was willing to replace multiple disks during a single surgery. My wife's American Airlines Blue Cross insurance plan would even pay for it.

I hired a specialized back consultant to guide me through the process. We had lunch one day in Orange County, California. But my pain was so intense, I couldn't focus on the conversation. In hindsight, I realized that the ADR surgery could've paralyzed me had it not worked.

Back pain affects many athletes. Wayne Gretzky famously had back problems all his days in the NHL. Because of back pain, Mario Lemieux left the Pittsburgh Penguins hockey team at the height of his amazing career. Roger Federer left tennis for one year while he rehabbed his own back. Tiger Woods suffered from back pain for 11 years and while taking opioids he was even arrested for DUI.

The most popular back therapy in tennis circles is physical therapy and spinal disk fusion. When PT doesn't work, an orthopedic surgeon will fuse the vertebrae together at the painful levels. The problem is that the back experiences intense levels of torque, pressure, and twist near the fusion point. This accelerates the degeneration above and below the spot of the fusion. Unless the patient stops sports entirely, the whole back eventually will need to be fused, causing nearly complete immobilization. I was unwilling to go that route.

Trigger Point Injections

My next step in the journey to becoming pain-free was to see a series of pain management anesthesiologists and pain doctors. Their mission was to treat the symptom, not cure the condition. At first, they would inject steroids into the areas of my back where I was suffering pain, hoping for a permanently good outcome. I did three of these, with relief lasting only a few days.

My next step was to allow these pain doctors to perform a series of radiofrequency ablations (RFAs). This procedure actually incorporated a hot probe into the nerves surrounding the pain point. The surgeon was unable to locate the specific sources of the pain. I found out later on that the nerves grow back eventually, which explains why the pain was alleviated only for a short period of time.

One doctor in Newport Beach, California, also a Palm Springs polo player, did two RFAs on my back with equally poor results. As a last-ditch effort, he prescribed an antidepressant called Cymbalta, thinking that perhaps the depression caused by the pain was itself causing more pain, and by alleviating my depression, the pain could be dissipated. This circular reasoning theory of pain, depression, more pain proved to be unhelpful. The antidepressant did not result in the pain being relieved.

In addition, unfortunately, one side effect of Cymbalta is insomnia. I was on this antidepressant for nearly a month. I slept only two or three fitful hours a night. The lack of sleep only made the back pain worse. I remember one night, before I had to give a speech in Philadelphia, staring at the ceiling at 4 a.m. contemplating a 9 a.m. speech. To counteract insomnia, I took Ambien. The first one didn't work, so I took another. That probably was the worst speech I had ever given. I couldn't remember my presentation and stammered throughout the program. The side effects of a drug I had hoped would dissipate back pain actually created more. The five cups of coffee only made me a wide-awake, drugged-up speaker! I stopped Cymbalta after that night, but the back pain persisted.

Still More Grief to Come?

One pain therapy method that worked was electrical stimulation, a TENS unit. (TENS stands for transcutaneous electrical nerve stimulation.) Six electrodes are put on your back via sticky glue pads. I would max out the pulsing electricity, allowing me to at least nod off. The unit had a timer. But often the electricity was so intense, my skin would burn. Other than narcotics, the unit was the only way to relieve my pain. I even played a tennis match with a TENS unit stuck on my back. Once an electrode fell off. I tried to replace it but only shocked myself. So much for physical activity during electrical therapy.

At that point, I bought a black foam roller. I would roll my back across it frequently during the day to relieve the discomfort. The store-bought roller was too big to carry in a suitcase. So I went to Home Depot and bought a 5-inch PVC pipe that did the trick. On one 14-hour flight to Hong Kong, my back was so jacked up that I rolled on the PVC pipe in the first-class galley. Several flight attendants were shocked and asked me to leave— but thankfully after I was done rolling on the floor.

I always carried a tennis ball when driving. I would put it behind my back and roll it up and down and side to side to alleviate the muscle spasms. Golf balls worked too. But being dependent on a tennis or golf ball is not the way to live one's life. Even that only decreased the pain from an 8 to a 7. The tennis ball was always my companion. I would've paid anything, done anything, traveled anywhere to get out of pain. I just didn't know how or what to do.

Light at the End of the Tunnel

One of my tennis friends, Eric Davidson, owner of the professional tennis team Orange County Breakers, had a problem with his rotator cuff. I saw him serve underhanded one day and asked what therapy he was getting. He mentioned stem cell treatment and a surgeon named Dr. Gaurav Goswami (yes, the coauthor of this book!). Eric was in the middle of therapy and did not have conclusive results yet. But I visited Dr. Goswami and asked for help. My condition was soft tissue ligaments in the thoracic area of the spine. I hoped to be a good candidate.

Dr. Goswami was thorough in his diagnosis and ordered a 3D CT scan to further look at my ribs and spine. He explained the complexity of my condition. Over the years, a lot of damage had occurred. Dr. Goswami explained the role stem cells play, how they are harvested, and how they could potentially regenerate ligament tissue. He also talked about the recovery period and what I could expect. Dr. Goswami warned me that the application of stem cells for my condition was rare and that multiple treatment sessions may be needed. I did not care. This was my last hope, my last resort. This was all I needed. I just wanted hope. I'd lived with so much pain for so long that any promise of a pain-free life was diminishing.

I'd been studying the platelet-rich plasma procedure for a few months. I'd even contacted a clinic in Chicago that promised PRP as a cure for any orthopedic condition. I was suspicious. I had friends who had PRP for tennis elbow, knee pain, wrist pain, and even cervical spine discomfort. One of the benefits of playing tennis is that you get to compare notes with other players who are injured. But PRP alone had mixed results.

I did my research on stem cell therapy. I knew stem cells were harvested from bone marrow and mesenchymal adipose tissue, and the PCP would be taken from my body's own blood. I also thought that stem cells could come from umbilical cord blood, which would be foreign to my body. Some clinics I researched would take my own bone marrow, store and enhance it over a few weeks in a foreign country, and then reinject it in my local problem area. But the procedure would be done outside the United States. This also made me uncomfortable, because these physicians were unable to practice in the United States.

I arrived at Dr. Goswami's office at 9 a.m. on the day of surgery. The nurse drew blood soon after. She led me to the surgical suite where Dr. Goswami harvested my cells. This took about 30 minutes. I was led to a comfortable chair outside the suite and chatted with the nurse as well as caught up on some emails.

After about three hours of spinning the cells, Dr. Goswami was able to concentrate my stem cells in a test tube. He put a fluoroscope over my back, using it to direct his injection to the right place. The stick was nearly pain-free, and it took only a few minutes. In fact, my biggest fear was the pain of the bone marrow extraction. I'd always heard this pain was among the most excruciating one could have. But besides a feeling of pressure and a click like a staple gun makes, there was nothing to it. Dr. Goswami gave me some natural anti-inflammatories including pomegranate juice. He also gave me two Vicodins to quell the discomfort for the next few days. That was it.

The next day, I was sore but not in pain. He told me to take it easy for the next six weeks avoiding tennis and working out at the gym. Otherwise, I could do any activity that I did before the surgery. No stitches were involved. This really wasn't like surgery. It was more like a procedure.

Post-procedure

A couple of weeks later, my wife and I went to the Barclays end-of-the-year pro tennis tournament in London, a tournament in which the top eight players in the world compete for millions of dollars in winnings. Before the tournament, we decided to take a side trip to Ireland. This included a bus excursion around the Ring of Kerry. The roads in Ireland are bumpy and inconsistent. The small tour bus I was in bounced like a trampoline. I was in the back seat when the bus hit a pothole. I went straight up into the ceiling and back down on my back, resulting in great pain. I was terrified that I might have destroyed all the great stem cell work Dr. Goswami did. In London, I visited a massage therapist who relaxed the tight muscles, alleviating most of the spasms. The tour bus bounce didn't harm the surgery in spite of my fears.

Three months after the surgery, the pain dropped from an 8 to a 4. I could play tennis again with the help of two anti-inflammatory pills. There was still discomfort, but I was back to hitting kick serves and moving much better. I was even quicker on the court than I had been. Before the treatment, I had told Dr.

Goswami that I would be happy if the pain level even dropped at all. Now seeing the promise of stem cell therapy, I wanted more. Nine months after the first procedure, I scheduled another.

In the meantime, my right knee was getting painful. It even collapsed a few times and was getting worse. Before the second procedure, Dr. Goswami suggested treating both my right and left knees to prevent further damage. We also decided to give another shot of stem cell therapy in my spinal thoracic 11 joint. Perhaps we could decrease the pain even more.

The second time was a charm. I haven't had any knee pain since the surgery. My back-pain level, which had gone from an 8 to a 4 after the first therapy, went from a 4 to a 2 after the second. This is more than I could've hoped for. I had been looking at life as a debilitating experience, with no sports, no activity, and a dependence on narcotics. My only hope was to live a life focused on avoiding pain instead of doing the things I love. Besides stem cell therapy, I tried physical therapy, pain management surgery, antidepressants, lidocaine pain patches, narcotics, and even electrical stimulation. Only stem cell therapy worked.

I still get sore muscles. But now I play tennis as if I were a teenager. I still get injured. But now I play tennis four times a week. I also play golf three times a week and do everything that I was prevented from doing for the past eight years.

What would you do to get out of pain? What would you do to get your life back? In my case, anything. My problem was that I didn't have the information or the options you have now by reading this book. I went through eight years of pain trying to find an answer. Learn from my mistakes and discovery.

I live in Portugal now, one month every quarter. One of my friends in the south of Portugal near Carvoeiro is a Lithuanian tennis player named Valentina. She is a lovely lady and had ankle surgery six months ago. Recently we spoke about how poor her outcome was. Her ankle is no better than it was before the surgery. I wish we could've talked before she went under the knife in Paris. She would've found that stem cell therapy is noninvasive and a natural first option before surgery. She may now be resigned to a painful ankle and a life with limited or no tennis.

But now you have options. Now you have alternatives. Now you have a choice. You can live without pain or debilitation. You now have the chance to try a therapy that likely will be a cure or at least significantly decrease your pain. There's no downside. This should be the first step before you consider orthopedic surgery. Stem cell therapy is an obvious choice for many. It can be for you too.

KEY TAKEAWAYS FROM KERRY

1. Never give up. Don't blindly accept an expert's recommendations. Keep exploring your options.
2. Do research and talk with others experiencing your condition.
3. Do not fall for fake treatments. Respect your body.

CHAPTER 15

The Future Is Now

Do not settle: Create your own healthy future.

Tying It All Together

After the discovery of penicillin, the application of stem cells is the most profound event in the history of medicine and healthcare. The future is already here. We have come full circle in medicine—from relying on drugs and surgeries, to using our own bodies to heal ourselves. For us to feel better, our cells need to heal. Foreign chemicals and unnecessary surgeries have not led us anywhere.

Nikola Tesla showed us how electricity and wireless communication work. It took Steve Jobs, Elon Musk, and a host of others to apply Tesla's theories to make life better. Similarly, understanding disease, illness, and injury at a cellular level over the last 20 years has opened the door to the clinical application of stem cells. But progress in medicine is always slower than in other fields. For the first time in healthcare, we're looking beyond just symptom management. We are trying to get to the root causes and fix those causes.

The term "stem cell" encompasses many different concepts. It includes various cells and a variety of treatments. Before therapy, it is critical to understand these differences. Our hope is that this book has helped you understand the world of stem cells. You now know a lot more about their benefits and limitations and what to look for in the future. There has been tremendous enthusiasm among patients and physicians, especially when it comes to treating certain challenging and sometimes incurable conditions that mainstream medicine often can't treat.

Why are so many patients seeking stem cell treatments? The answer to this question is that people are likely to seek stem cell treatments:

- When mainstream medicine offers no cure
- When mainstream medicine fails
- When mainstream medicine offers treatments with toxic side effects or risky surgery

You don't want your quality of life to suffer. You have limited time on this planet. Hospitals and doctors' offices are the last place you should be spending your precious time.

Responsibility to Be Safe

With anything new comes responsibility. This responsibility is a duty to prove that stem cells are effective. This includes a duty for us to take collective responsibility as a society to help integrate stem cells into mainstream medicine. Stem cell treatments are going to require a physician who understands not only your specific problem but also your whole body. At no other time in medicine has it been more important to view the patient as a whole instead of just focusing on one specific condition. You will also have to assume responsibility. No treatment can work unless your body has the capacity to heal. The body will heal if you maintain and take care of it.

Your own stem cells have been the single most important discovery of this century. The ability now to harvest, collect, and isolate your own stem cells opens up a whole new door of opportunity. This is especially true when we are treating joint pain, sports injuries, and back pain. Your own mesenchymal stem cells belong to the same family of cells that form cartilage, meniscus, bone, muscles, and ligaments. These mesenchymal stem cells can be collected from your body sources such as blood, bone marrow, fat, muscle, and joint lining. These cells require no modification in the laboratory to help repair your damage, because they are like-minded and belong to the same family of tissues seen in your joints and spine. Most treatments are done using the same-day, same-sitting protocol in order to give you fresh cells. No storage or mixing with chemicals is involved. There is no fear of rejection by your body. No risk of introducing any foreign disease. No risk of developing tumors.

In addition to stem cells, your blood provides platelets. When isolated, platelet-rich plasma contains 10 anti-inflammatory and growth-promoting factors. Think of PRP as an excellent fertilizer that helps stimulate the growth of your stem cells.

Your own stem cells can help 90% of the conditions you may suffer. Your own stem cells are safest for your body. You cannot ask for a more natural treatment. This is the single most important incentive to take care of your body. If your body is healthy, you can tap into your own stem cells anytime you need them.

Stem Cells and Sports Injury

CASE STUDY: **NICK**

Nick is a 23-year-old professional boxer and burgeoning MMA fighter with a 3–0 record. All his victories so far were knockouts (KOs). During the last fight, his knee took a beating. It felt extremely painful and sore. He set up a meeting with his surgeon, who recommended arthroscopic surgery. Hungry for his next opponent, Nick underwent surgery and the required rehab for 10 weeks. Nick recovered well from the surgery but was unable to start practicing for three months after. He was in considerable pain. While he could take the discomfort, it was his inability to practice that was becoming worrisome. He was anxious to get back in the ring and further build upon his professional record. Another three months went by, and Nick was unable to put much weight on his knee. He was unable to practice full steam. His surgeon said there was significant scar tissue buildup. He may need another surgery to clean up the joint. This just didn't sound right to Nick. He was frustrated. He was raised by a mother who believed in a holistic approach with a lot of natural therapy. She advised him to seek other opinions and options prior to even considering a second surgery.

Nick did his research. He called other doctors specializing in managing knee injuries. He came across a little-known physician focused on regenerative cell therapy. Nick flew down to see the doctor. He underwent a thorough clinical and imaging assessment including movements associated with his chosen sport. Along with the damage inside the knee, Nick had also suffered injury to his lateral collateral ligament (LCL) that supports the outside part of the knee.

Over the next two months, Nick underwent three rounds of treatments using his own stem cells. They were harvested and injected back fresh on the same day. This was important to Nick. Being a professional athlete, he did not want any foreign substance in his body. He also did not want to take a chance with stem cells that were biologically altered in the laboratory. His own stem cells were injected targeting both the inside of his knee and the outside ligaments. Each treatment lasted about three hours. Nick walked out with no stitches, just Band-Aids. Three months after his first treatment, Nick was back in the ring practicing. Within six months Nick was fighting again. Nick has since participated in two professional fights. His record now stands at 5–0 with five KOs.

Ongoing Research

Tremendous amounts of research are being done in the world of stem cells. Initial enthusiasm was focused on embryonic stem cells. These may be capable of developing into any cell type and organ system. However, the risk of introducing foreign material into your body, not to mention sacrificing human life to procure these cells, is not the direction to go. Your own cells can be studied carefully in a laboratory and then programmed to develop into specific different cells based on your needs. Your body is teeming with your own stem cells. For certain conditions, they can be safely collected and used the same day to help your body regenerate and repair. As we have stated before, your own stem cells are safest since they belong to you. Other sources of cells are umbilical cord, placenta, and amnion, all derived when these sources are no longer needed by a newborn baby. There is no loss of human life or a threat to the infant. How these foreign birth-related cells are collected, cleaned, and ultimately prepared for use in your body requires careful study. Currently, there are no standardized methods for completing these steps. One has to be extremely careful. Before claims can be made, much more needs to be learned to fully understand the characteristics of the different types of stem cells.

No matter the source, we are just at the tip of the stem cell iceberg. We should all be extremely prudent in our approach. The future indeed holds great promise!

For example, think about the child born with cerebral palsy or with a developmental abnormality or some congenital disease. With certain conditions, children don't live past their teenage years. Think about children suffering from type 1 diabetes, whose bodies cannot produce insulin. Or think about the high school teenager whose budding career in sports is ruined by an injury. This will rob the teen of a sport that brings him or her joy.

Think about a parent, uncle, or aunt paralyzed in an accident. These folks may never again do what they love. They may be unable to ride a motorcycle, play golf, or travel to see the grandkids. Or consider the life of a mechanic who after years of hard work and labor is about to lose his vision due to macular degeneration. He won't be able to see his children or grandchildren enjoy the fruits of his labor.

These situations can take a heavy toll, not only on the patients but also on their caregivers and families. We are making daily progress to find stem cells able to help each of these patients. There is hope.

Other than the conditions discussed in their individual chapters, let's look at some other rare applications of stem cells.

Stem Cells and Cancer

CASE STUDY: **DIEGO**

Diego is a kid who absolutely loves baseball. Even at age 11, he takes practice time very seriously. Both parents supported his passion and proved it by being his taxi to different league matches. One day on the field, Diego started feeling intense pain in his hip. After a few hours, the pain subsided. He did not think much of it. A few weeks later, he had even more intense pain in his back, in his pelvis, and again in his hip area. His parents felt he was playing too much and should cut down baseball time.

After a few days, Diego noticed his gums hurt as he brushed his teeth. He was also feeling lethargic. For the first time, he had no desire to get back on the field. His parents took him to a doctor, who ordered blood tests for Diego. The next day the physician told the parents that Diego should be immediately seen by a specialist. Diego was diagnosed with blood cancer. His bone marrow was producing excessive amounts of one particular cell. The diagnosis devastated the family. Diego had no clue about what all this meant.

Over the next few days, more tests were done. Diego started feeling pain just getting out of bed. He missed games. He developed a fever and cough. It was recommended that Diego undergo chemotherapy. The chemo medications had severe side effects. He became weak, and nausea from the chemotherapy was so severe that, along with having headaches, he rarely slept. Six months after starting chemo, Diego's blood counts were not improving, and his bones were still very painful. Chemotherapy had killed the bad cells in his body. But Diego needed those to be replaced with new, healthy cells that could produce normal ones.

In other words, he needed a stem cell transplant. Diego underwent the procedure. After a few months, he started regaining strength. It's been seven years now, and Diego is cancer-free.

Stem Cells and Sickle Cell Disease

Sickle cell disease is an inherited blood disorder that most often, but not always, affects people of African descent. Hemoglobin is a protein in your red blood cells that carries oxygen. Sickle cell is a genetic defect that alters the structure of the hemoglobin.

The defect causes red blood cells to lose their normal round shape and become deformed. The new shape resembles a sickle, hence the name of the condition. These deformed cells can then block blood flow in different organs, causing pain, organ damage, and even stroke. There is no available cure for sickle cell disease.

CASE STUDY: JOHN

John suffered from sickle cell all his life. He battled infections and multiple hospitalizations. Now in his 30s, John constantly lived in fear that his next crisis could be fatal. He was desperate to find a more robust treatment. His doctor called one day and wondered if John wished to enroll in a clinical trial where stem cells would be involved. Stem cells would be collected from a normal healthy donor who had been matched to John. John received a short course of chemotherapy that destroyed his abnormal cells. The new stem cells were then infused into his body. It's been three years since John's treatment. Since then, he's been hospitalized only once.

Stem Cells and Cerebral Palsy

Cerebral palsy is a lifelong physical disability involving limitation of movement or motor function. This usually starts in early childhood and is due to brain cell damage. There is no cure. The degree of disability can vary from needing assistance with walking to being so debilitated that the sufferer is completely wheelchair-bound. Other associated problems such as pain, intellectual disability, seizures, inability to talk or hear, blindness, and sleeplessness can also occur. A variety of stem cells are currently being studied. Preliminary results show improvement in motor function. The benefits may not be seen in all patients. How long these benefits will last is equally unknown.

The Stem Cell Revolution Is Here

The patients described above were desperate. They were inching toward death. Stem cell treatments gave them hope for a cure. These treatments represent a revolution that is starting from the ground up. When your neighbor can be healed from a simple stem cell knee injection, why would you want to be subjected to surgery and prolonged rehab? Before treatment, that neighbor was probably in pain and unable to walk. Yet you likely saw her six weeks later walking the dogs for miles. If you knew all that, wouldn't you be curious about her cure? Wouldn't that be an interesting question to ask your doctor, insurance provider, or local regulatory agency?

Regulators and Insurance Companies Need to Catch Up

Regulatory organizations and insurance companies will have to demonstrate an open mind to understand what stem cells really are and the variables involved. Unfortunately, when it comes to your own stem cells, there is no lobby likely to help. Even though they may be the safest option, you might be forced to use other, harmful, treatments. Regulatory bodies and health insurance companies have to understand the science behind the use of your own stem cells. They will need to work with scientists, physicians, and patients to develop a regulatory framework that will help you utilize the power of your stem cells. Sooner or later, if we do not implement these changes, both on a personal level and at a societal level, we will again have to learn some hard lessons.

Medicine doesn't always grow from university-led medical research breakthroughs. Leadership is overestimated. As noted above, real change comes from the ground up. We are all leaders. You are the leader. Take command of your body, your mind, and your actions. Don't wait for someone else to step up for great change to follow. That is a smokescreen. If you have a medical condition and current options don't make sense, don't acquiesce. Through research, educate yourself about stem cells. Get opinions and make a commitment to asking questions until you find answers. We often misdirect our priorities. People spend more time researching their next vacation than their treatments. Personal responsibility is very important if we are to maximize our life and extend the promise of a healthy and more productive life to future generations.

Live well!

SUMMARY

The term "stem cells" is used to describe many types of processes and treatments. Two patients can have so-called stem cell treatments, and yet the entire process may be completely different. So can the outcomes. Understand the role stem cells are likely to play in your particular condition. Separate hype from fact. We recommend these top five questions to ask yourself when seeking stem cell treatment:

1. What type of stem cells am I getting?
2. How many live stem cells am I getting?
3. How will they be delivered into my body?
4. How many stem cell treatments will I need?
5. What should success from my stem cell procedure look like?

Acknowledgments

This book would not have seen the light of the day without the support of the following individuals. Thanks to Dan Strutzel, our agent, for believing in this project. Sandra Deleon for keeping the medical practice afloat when the writer overtook the physician. Ruby Quinones and Katarina Kiesselbach for providing follow-up on many patients whose case histories have been discussed. Kimberly Conroy for transcribing portions when our fingers got too tired. Much appreciation is due to our publisher, Mary Glenn, and her team at Humanix for taking up this extremely timely topic.

Index

About the Authors

Gaurav Goswami, M.D., M.S., DABIR, is a surgeon and minimally invasive specialist practicing in Newport Beach California. Dr. Goswami has spent the last decade developing protocols in advanced regenerative treatments. Founded by Dr Goswami, The Goswami Clinic offers treatment methods aimed at tissue preservation. The clinic has focused on utilizing the power of your own cells to heal many conditions related to overuse of muscles and joints. We believe no matter the age or level, there is an athlete in all of us. Physical mobility along with a sound mind are extremely important for our patients to enjoy their life. At the Goswami clinic we recognize this and aim to achieve functional results for our patients—outcomes that help our patients perform in their daily life or chosen sports. While mainstream medicine (at its best) has only provided occasional symptomatic control, at The Goswami Clinic we take treatments to the next level—not just pain relief but true healing, regeneration, and repair. Our motto is "Don't just return to play, return to perform." Along with clinical care, Dr. Goswami is involved in training and research to further advance the science of regenerative and restorative medicine. Dr. Goswami is an Assistant Professor at Western Health

Sciences University Southern California. He can be reached at TheGoswamiClinic.com

Kerry Johnson, MBA, Ph.D., is an international speaker and bestselling author. He is an adjunct professor and has written 12 books including, *Mastering the Game, Why Smart People Make Dumb Mistakes with Their Money*, and *New Mindset, New Results*. In the 1970s he played professional tennis on the International Grand Prix Tennis Tour. To hear Kerry speak live, click on www.KerryJohnson.com.

Improve Memory and Sharpen Your Mind

Misplacing your keys, forgetting someone's name at a party, or coming home from the market without the most important item — these are just some of the many common memory slips we all experience from time to time.

Most of us laugh about these occasional memory slips, but for some, it's no joke. Are these signs of dementia, or worse, Alzheimer's? Dr. Garry Small will help dissuade those fears and teach you practical strategies and exercises to sharpen your mind in his breakthrough book, *2 Weeks To A Younger Brain*.

This book will show that it only takes two weeks to form new habits that bolster cognitive abilities and help stave off or even reverse brain aging.

If you commit only 14 days to *2 Weeks To A Younger Brain*, you will reap noticeable results. During that brief period, you will have learned the secrets of keeping your brain young for the rest of your life.

Claim Your FREE OFFER Now!

Claim your **FREE** copy of *2 Weeks To A Younger Brain* — a $19.99 value — today with this special offer. Just cover $4.95 for shipping & handling.

Plus, you will receive a 3-month risk-free trial subscription to *Dr. Gary Small's Mind Health Report*. Renowned brain expert and psychiatrist Gary Small, M.D., fills every issue of *Mind Health Report* with the latest advancements and breakthrough techniques for improving & enhancing your memory, brain health, and longevity. **That's a $29 value, yours FREE!**

Allergy-Proof Your Life

Natural Remedies for Allergies That Work!

Inside *Allergy-Proof Your Life*:

- ✓ **What You Should Never, Ever Eat if You Suffer From Allergies**
- ✓ Dangers and Limitations of Common Allergy Medications
- ✓ **Top Foods & Nutrients to Help You Fight Allergies**
- ✓ The Gut-Allergy Connection Your Doctor Won't Tell You About
- ✓ **And Much More . . .**

Claim Your FREE OFFER Now!

Claim your **FREE** copy of *Allergy-Proof Your Life* — a **$24.99 value** — today with this special offer. Just cover $4.95 for shipping & handling.

Plus, you will receive a bonus **FREE** report — *Over-the-Counter Health Hazards* — from one of America's foremost holistic physicians, David Brownstein, M.D.

We'll also send you a 3-month risk-free trial subscription to **Dr. David Brownstein's Natural Way to Health** which provides you with the most recent insights on emerging natural treatments along with the best of safe conventional medical care.

"*Allergy-Proof Your Life* is a great resource for all allergy sufferers. It helps you discover the underlying causes of your allergies, so you can heal them once and for all."
— **Dr. Brownstein, M.D.**

Get Your FREE Copy of *Allergy-Proof* TODAY!
Newsmax.com/Stem

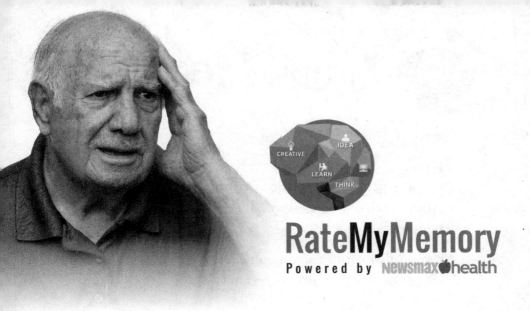

RateMyMemory

Powered by newsmax health

Normal Forgetfulness?
Something More Serious?

You forget things — names of people, where you parked your car, the place you put an important document, and so much more. Some experts tell you to dismiss these episodes.

"Not so fast," says Dr. Gary Small, director of the UCLA Longevity Center, medical researcher, professor of psychiatry, and the *New York Times* best-selling author of *2 Weeks to a Younger Brain*.

Dr. Small says that most age-related memory issues are normal but sometimes can be a warning sign of future cognitive decline.

Now Dr. Small has created the online **RateMyMemory Test** — allowing you to easily assess your memory strength in just a matter of minutes.

It's time to begin your journey of making sure your brain stays healthy and young! **It takes just 2 minutes!**

Test Your Memory Today:
MemoryRate.com/Stem

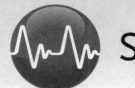 # Simple **Heart Test**

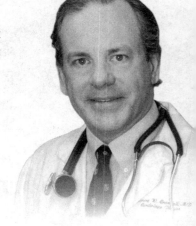

FACT:

▶ Nearly half of those who die from heart attacks each year never showed prior symptoms of heart disease.

▶ If you suffer cardiac arrest outside of a hospital, you have just a 7% chance of survival.

Don't be caught off guard. Know your risk now.

TAKE THE TEST NOW ...

Renowned cardiologist **Dr. Chauncey Crandall** has partnered with **Newsmaxhealth.com** to create a simple, easy-to-complete, online test that will help you understand your heart attack risk factors. Dr. Crandall is the author of the #1 best-seller *The Simple Heart Cure: The 90-Day Program to Stop and Reverse Heart Disease.*

Take Dr. Crandall's Simple Heart Test — it takes just 2 minutes or less to complete — it could save your life!

Discover your risk now.

- **Where you score on our unique heart disease risk scale**
- **Which of your lifestyle habits really protect your heart**
- **The true role your height and weight play in heart attack risk**
- Little-known conditions that impact heart health
- **Plus much more!**

SimpleHeartTest.com/Stem